Advance Praise for the Second Edition of *Overcoming Secondary Stress in Medical and Nursing Practice* . . .

"Dr. Robert Wicks and Dr. Gloria Donnelly's updated book provides timely guidance and invaluable, concrete strategies to better understand and prevent stress and the cycle of burnout. This book should be on all healthcare providers' list of required readings as they prepare to face the rewards and challenges of our ever-changing healthcare environment."

Patrick C. Auth, PhD, PA-C, DFAAPA 2017
Physician Assistant Education Association,
Leadership Development Awardee

"I prescribe this go-to resource for healing professionals in Medicine and Nursing who entered into practice psychologically healthy and now feel damaged. It's a life jacket for all who are drowning in unrelenting stress wrought by COVID-19, the current machinery of corporate healthcare delivery, and individual life circumstances. Wicks and Donnelly expertly help readers to gain perspective into their unique situations and start their personal healing journey. If your passion for healthcare is fading fast, reach for this book to become revitalized."

Linda Laskowski-Jones, MS, APRN, ACNS-BC,
CEN, NEA-BC, FAWM, FAAN
Editor in Chief, Nursing2020 Journal:
The Peer-Reviewed Journal of Clinical Excellence
Health, Learning, Research & Practice

"Burnout" of healthcare professionals preceded the COVID-19 pandemic. The pandemic has brought the problem "front and center". *Overcoming Secondary Stress in Medical and Nursing Practice* is a beautifully written book; a must read not only for all healthcare providers and their employers, but their relatives. This compassionate, concise text provides a clear blueprint for understanding why stress is a pervasive problem for medical and nursing professionals along with strategic solutions for prevention, endurance, and resilience.

Julie H. Levison, MD, MPhil, MPH, FACP
Assistant Professor in Medicine, Harvard Medical School
Division of General Internal Medicine and the Morgan Institute
Massachusetts General Hospital

"We are living in unprecedented times. Living through a pandemic, health providers have had to radically alter how they practice, for example, learning how to do telehealth overnight. This power-packed book should be read by all health care providers, whether they are administrators, educators, researchers or frontline staff. Secondary stress confronts us all and this book assists health providers to manage such stress."

Al Rundio, PhD, DNP, RN, APRN, NEA-BC, FAArN
Vice President for Scholarly Advancement/
Co-Editor-In-Chief for Practice
Journal of Interprofessional Education & Practice
National Academies of Practice

Reviews of First Edition of *Overcoming Secondary Stress in Medical and Nursing Practice . . .*

"...brief, to the point, and practical...a very valuable resource for any health professional working in today's healthcare arena."

(5 Stars—Highest Rating)—*Doody's*

"Reading Dr. Robert Wicks' *Overcoming Secondary Stress in Medical and Nursing Practice* is both a personal and professional pleasure . . . I particularly enjoyed completing the Medical-Nursing Secondary Stress Questionnaire and using my answers as a 'springboard' for further self-reflection and as the basis for developing my own self-care protocol. I would urge physicians, nurses, and other health care professionals to keep a copy of this wonderful resource with them at all times; I certainly intend to do so!"

Anne Belcher, PhD, RN, AOCN, FAAN
Senior Associate Dean for Academic Affairs
The Johns Hopkins University School of Nursing

"The technical and organizational pressures on those providing medical care today are often overwhelming. This book is a much-needed practical aid which can equip the caregiver with the insights for coping successfully with caregiver stresses."

Edmund D. Pellegrino, MD
Professor Emeritus of Medicine and Medical Ethics
Georgetown University

"This power-packed book is a must-read for all professionals who are responsible for the health care of others . . . [it] provides insightful and practical self-care strategies to help us take better care of ourselves so we can be better at what we do and sustain our abilities to do so."

Ruth McCorkle, PhD, FAAN
The Florence S. Wald Professor of Nursing
Director, Center for Excellence in Chronic Illness Care
Yale University School of Nursing

Overcoming Secondary Stress
in Medical and Nursing Practice

Overcoming Secondary Stress
IN MEDICAL AND NURSING PRACTICE

A Guide to Professional Resilience and Personal Well-Being

SECOND EDITION

ROBERT J. WICKS AND
GLORIA F. DONNELLY

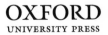

OXFORD
UNIVERSITY PRESS

OXFORD
UNIVERSITY PRESS

Oxford University Press is a department of the University of Oxford. It furthers
the University's objective of excellence in research, scholarship, and education
by publishing worldwide. Oxford is a registered trade mark of Oxford University
Press in the UK and certain other countries.

Published in the United States of America by Oxford University Press
198 Madison Avenue, New York, NY 10016, United States of America.

© Oxford University Press 2021

First Edition published in 2005
Second Edition published in 2021

Library of Congress Cataloging-in-Publication Data
Names: Wicks, Robert J., author. | Donnelly, Gloria F. author.
Title: Overcoming secondary stress in medical and nursing practice :
a guide to professional resilience and personal well-being / by Robert
J. Wicks and Gloria F. Donnelly.
Description: Second edition. | New York : Oxford University Press, [2021] |
Includes bibliographical references and index.
Identifiers: LCCN 2020036332 (print) | LCCN 2020036333 (ebook) |
ISBN 9780197547243 (paperback) | ISBN 9780197547267 (epub)
Subjects: LCSH: Physicians—Job stress. | Nurses—Job stress. | Medical
personnel—Job stress. | Physicians—Mental health. | Nurses—Mental
health. | Medical personnel—Mental health. | Burn out
(Psychology) —Prevention. | Self-care, Health. | Resilience (Personality
trait) | Stress management.
Classification: LCC R707 .W535 2021 (print) | LCC R707 (ebook) |
DDC 610.6901/9—dc23
LC record available at https://lccn.loc.gov/2020036332
LC ebook record available at https://lccn.loc.gov/2020036333

9 8 7 6 5 4 3 2 1

Printed by LSC Communications, United States of America

My mother-in-law, Dorothy Barry, believed that as a profession nursing is both honorable and dedicated to what is good in this world. Two of her daughters, my wife, Michaele, and my sister-in-law, Deborah Kibble, took their mother's beliefs to heart and became nurses. And so, it is to the three of them that I dedicate this book.

Robert J. Wicks

I dedicate this book to those practicing medicine and nursing who have worked heroically and tirelessly to care for patients throughout the COVID-19 pandemic.

Gloria F. Donnelly

Contents

Foreword

It is through humor that I first become acquainted with then Dean Gloria Donnelly when she was performing standup comedy to benefit her college at Drexel University where I also taught. I immediately concluded it was a good idea to get to know this academic leader and scholar who had a way with humor. It was a meeting of the minds, so to speak, as I am continually impressed with her practical insights. Her collaboration with Robert Wicks, the renowned psychologist and author working at the intersection of psychology and spirituality and the prevention of secondary stress, was bound to yield an invaluable contribution to the health care professional well-being literature. Forgiving oneself, greater self-awareness of secondary stress, exercises that reduce angst, and enhance well-being are integral parts of this important book. Read it thoroughly, apply its lessons, and keep it on a shelf nearby so you can refer to it in those emotional emergencies that are likely to crop up in the busy life of a health care professional. Primary and secondary stressors are sure to come to the health professional; be prepared to handle them effectively and take the preventive measures to make sure they do not turn into something worse. I know that there are several times in my career in medical practice, medical research, and academic executive leadership roles spanning more than four decades when I would have found this book a handy guide for weathering the vicissitudes of a medical career in challenging times.

Wicks and Donnelly make use of vignettes, provide instructive tables and personalized self-care protocols that by altering perspectives away from the reflexive ones, health care practitioners can reduce reactivity, anger, moral, and emotional distress. The authors provide techniques for accomplishing this including mindfulness practices that are associated with Buddhism or Christianity as well as making use of humor, participating in a weekend spiritual retreat, engaging with loved ones, exercise, journaling, and many more techniques. Such features as the Secondary Stress Self-Awareness Questionnaire help personalize the material for the reader and make the recommendations all that more useful.

Overcoming Secondary Stress in Medical and Nursing Practice is an extraordinarily timely and highly practical book addressing health care professional burnout, its prevention and effective management in the time of COVID-19. It should be a crucial addition to the library of every medical professional because it provides important advice on how to avoid the secondary stress of being a health professional, its emotional and moral distress. Burnout in the medical professions was a substantial hazard before the pandemic because of the corporate takeover of health care as well as the computerization of medical practice and the changing roles of the medical professions in society. (I described the cultural and social foundational factors for these changes in *Ethos of Medicine in Postmodern America: Philosophical, Cultural and Social Considerations* [Lexington Books, Rowman and Littlefield, 2015]).

Today in the wake of the pandemic, close to half of health care professionals are reporting symptoms of depression. A meta-analysis published just before the pandemic began indicated that physicians have an increased risk of suicide compared to other professionals (RR 1.44) and female physicians (RR1.9) had the greatest risk.[1] Nurses have an increased risk of suicide as well (RR1.39).[2] So the stakes for reducing and overcoming secondary stress are very high indeed. Wicks and Donnelly show that a great deal can be done to counter the harmful effects of secondary stress in medical and nursing practice. Dealing effectively with secondary stress can be literally a matter of life or death. Of course, there can be much suffering well short of suicide that needs to be reduced or prevented so that these professions can be practiced and enjoyed in our times.

We do not get to choose the era we live in, so these pressing issues on the nature of health care practice today must be addressed effectively.

The well-being of those practicing these important professions including physicians, nurses, physician assistants, respiratory therapists, social workers, and many other types of health care practitioners is of paramount importance as the effectiveness of health care is dependent on well-adjusted practitioners. This volume will help its readers accomplish that adjustment to the new normal and help them thrive in our challenging health care environment.

Arnold R. Eiser, MD, MACP
Adjunct Senior Fellow, Leonard Davis Institute
Perelman School of Medicine
University of Pennsylvania
Professor Emeritus, Drexel University College of Medicine

References

1. Dutheil F, Aubert C, Pereira B, et al. Suicide among physicians and health-care workers: A systematic review and meta-analysis. *PLoS One.* 2019;14(12):e0226361

2. Davidson JE, Proudfoot J, Lee K, Terterian G, Zisook S. A longitudinal analysis of nurse suicide in the United States (2005–2016) with recommendations for action. *Worldviews on Evidence-Based Nursing.* 2020;17(1):6–15.

Reaching Out . . . Without Being Pulled Down

Remaining Passionate in the Fields of Medicine and Nursing, a Guide to Personal and Professional Well-Being for Physicians, Physician Assistants, and Nurses

Objectives of the Introduction

- Understand the meaning and effects of secondary stress.
- Recognize how culture, environment, and the demands of modern healthcare lead to secondary stress in health professionals.
- Appreciate that no matter how healthy you are, stress is part and parcel of involvement in the practice of medicine and nursing.
- Explore strategies for preventing, limiting, and learning from the occurrences of secondary stress such as (a) heightened awareness of personal, interpersonal, and environmental stressors; (b) the necessity of developing a self-care protocol; (c) ways to strengthen one's inner life; and (d) strategies to increase self-knowledge as a way of enhancing personal and professional well-being.

These mountains that you are carrying, you were only supposed to climb.

—Najwa Zebian

The end of the inner-city emergency department 12-hour shift approaches. Several staff gravitate to the lounge to gather themselves and to have a cup of coffee to fuel the drive home. Karen, an emergency room (ER) staff nurse and Kevin, a physician assistant share a small table. The COVID-19 pandemic has been raging for the past several weeks. To keep her husband and two young children safe, Karen convinced them to live with the in-laws until the crisis passes. In addition to working as an ER staff nurse, Karen is attending an online program to earn her master's in nursing degree. The pace of work during the epidemic has taken its toll on her schoolwork, on relationships, on everything. Kevin completed his physician assistant program six months ago and never imagined this work intensity. He is living temporarily in a motel near the hospital to conserve his energy and protect his family. Jack, a veteran ER resident physician, enters the lounge, plops in a chair, and stares into space. "Mrs. Alverez just died. I just got off the phone with her family. They begged to visit, but the rule is the rule. It was gut wrenching for me to say 'no.'"

Tears stream down Karen's face, "I am just numb, pretty much running on automatic pilot, which is how I get through the shift. I do not remember half the patients that I care for or what I do for them. In one sense I am grateful that family cannot visit and that you are making those calls, and I feel so guilty about that but I cannot imagine the added pressure of dealing with family when so many patients are so critically ill and close to death. I love taking care of patients especially in the ER but never imagined this—like being at war." Jack and Kevin nod in agreement. Kevin questions his career choice, "I did not sign on for war!" They sit in silence staring at the table.

This book is written for those who practice medicine (physicians and physician assistants) and those who practice nursing. There is no more compelling time for physicians, physician assistants, and nurses to examine the experience of secondary stress than on the heels of the COVID-19 pandemic. This second edition of *Overcoming Secondary Stress in Medical and Nursing Practice* is designed to alert those who practice medicine and nursing to the sources, acuity, and chronicity of secondary stress (the pressures experienced in reaching out to others) in the clinical environment; to the context in which secondary stressors are most likely to occur; to environmental conditions that provoke secondary stress; and to ways that strengthen the inner lives and overall health of those in the healing professions. This book is also written for leaders and administrators who can initiate the changes in health care systems needed to manage stress and prevent burnout among direct care clinicians. Overcoming secondary stress is a collective effort by individual practitioners and those who create the environmental conditions of health care delivery. In the modern health care setting, the information in this book is not simply desirable; it is essential for one's personal and professional well-being.

The demands of modern health care on those who practice medicine and nursing are cumulatively extreme and include

- heavy clinical caseloads with rising inpatient acuity as procedural care continues to revert to same day or outpatient services.
- demands to learn new technologies including what seems like endless documentation of care processes.
- demanding patients and families now called *consumers* who do not understand the complexity of clinical care.
- patient satisfaction measurement systems that can be indicting to practitioners and that can affect reimbursement and compensation.
- unreasonable expectations of employers who continue to deal with a "more with less" reimbursement system.
- unreasonable or uncivil colleagues who catalyze hostile work environments.
- self-doubt and grief that often accompanies a review of ones' decisions on behalf of patients.

If there is an apt proverb for the articulated and unspoken demands many people make of medical and nursing professionals today, it surely must be the Yiddish one: "Sleep faster. . . . We need the pillows!"

Christina Maslach, the social psychologist and noted authority on burnout, recounts her invitation by the government of Sweden to examine the effects of stress segments of the workforce. Government leaders were concerned with what they termed crises in workplaces leading to resignations and shortages in some fields. As Maslach[1] recounts,

it turned out that there's a social insurance system for everybody who works in Sweden. If you are going out on sick leave or some sort of disability, and you leave your job, they'll pay your salary for up to a year and a half. They put you in treatment for whatever it is you need, and after the year and a half, you go back to your original job.

What they were seeing was this sharp increase in the number of people going out on sick leave from the healthcare field and from IT. They were particularly concerned because when they looked at the diagnosis, it was severe clinical depression work-related only. They'd say, "It sounds like burnout, that it's depression but only work-related." As my colleagues and I, looked at the data and we saw that "Well, actually, we think maybe burnout happened upstream, before this. You now have a problem with severe clinical depression, and that's what you've got to treat, but there was probably a warning sign that people weren't paying attention to, or didn't know about, earlier on."

Maslach's insights and Sweden's concerns ring true in different ways for all health care professionals today. Professional organizations such as the American Medical Association, the American Academy of Physician Assistants, and the American Nurses' Association are addressing the same phenomenon observed in Sweden in 2019 by developing standards and programs that will contain the effects of secondary stress on their members. The American Medical Association features continuing education modules for physicians to prevent burnout and address well-being through its Stepsforward program.[2] The Accreditation Review Commission on Education for the Physician Assistant has added a criterion to their national standards addressing work stress and self-care that all physician assistant programs must address in educational programs. Standard B2.20 for physician assistant programs is, "The curriculum must include instruction about provider personal wellness including prevention of: a) impairment and b) burnout."[3] The American Nurses Association is working to ensure Healthy Work Environments for nurses focusing on reasonable staffing, nurse health and safety, and prevention of nurse abuse including incivility, bullying, and violence.[4] These professional organizations are working to change the culture of modern health care, which is, at least, partially responsible for secondary stress and burnout among direct care providers.

The Culture of Health Care

The COVID-19 pandemic has exposed many stress-inducing shortcomings of the health care system such as lack of preparedness, limited clinical capacity and protective equipment for clinical staff, and an ethic of doing more with less, highlighting the risks incurred in everyday practice. And there is more. Surveys of physicians, physician assistants, and nurses continue to highlight the negative impact of work culture and conditions on physical and mental health. The culture of health care is multileveled, including national trends such as the corporatization of health care, for-profit health care systems, the computerization of practice, and the maldistribution of services that lead to health disparities. There are also the cultures of specific work environments, framed by national trends, that create either healthy or toxic work environments. A 2015 Medscape survey[5] of U.S. physicians reported that the top four leading causes of burnout were (a) too many bureaucratic tasks leading to loss of autonomy, (b) too many hours at work leading to extreme work life balance issues, (c) insufficient income related to declining reimbursements, and (d) an increasing computerization of health care leading to less facetime with patients, a phenomenon that Eiser[6] terms "the silicon cage."

Coplan et al.'s 2018 study of burnout, job satisfaction, and stress levels of physician assistants reported similar findings to the Medscape survey of physicians.[7] The highest rated factors contributing to stress included (a) too many work hours, (b) income not high enough, (c) too many bureaucratic and administrative tasks, and (d) feeling like a cog in a wheel.

In 2013, the American Nurses Association launched a Health Risk Appraisal as part of its Healthy Nurse–Healthy Nation initiative.[8] Three years of data from the survey reports of 13,500 registered nurses revealed that (a) 82 percent reported experiencing workplace stress including bullying and aggression particularly from peers rather than supervisors; (b) 25 percent had been physically attacked by patients or visitors; (c) more than 40 percent cited physical stressors such as lifting, prolonged standing, needlesticks, and exposure to blood borne pathogens; and (d) respondents also reported a drop in sleep hours and failure to eat a reasonably healthy diet.

The results of these surveys provide incontrovertible evidence that many health professionals are at risk. In their contact with patients, not only may healing professionals contract a physical disease, they are in even greater danger of being "infected" psychologically. Secondary stress, *the pressure that results from reaching out to others in need*, is a constant and continuous reality for physicians, physician assistants, and nurses. And, considering the culture of health care and disruptions such as the pandemic, it is a situation to be reckoned with in new ways.

The stakes are now so high for health care professionals that the potential for developing such psychological problems as emotional blunting on the one hand or extreme affectivity on the other is quite great. Many deny their own emotional needs as a survival mechanism or keep silent in environments of turmoil. However, physicians, physician assistants, and nurses often follow the implicit advice to protect themselves by not allowing themselves to feel too much emotion.

Professionals, who have committed their lives to caring for others, are overwhelmed by frustrations and loss of perspective as stressors of the health care environment and its multiple cultures and demands bear down. Changes in practice driven by unreasonable quests for efficiency and profit, inequity that produces health disparities, societal and world instability as in pandemics, physical demands, and self-induced pressures fueled by unhealthy work environments make up only part of a psychological and physical combustible mixture. Therefore, not addressing these conditions is not only foolish; it is also dangerous to the well-being of talented, caring, and hitherto emotionally healthy persons working in the healing professions—the audience for whom this book is written.

This Book's Framework

Overcoming Secondary Stress in Medical and Nursing Practice is a book designed to sit prominently on your desk for quick access. Randomly opening to any page in the book will convey the message that you are not alone and that you have and can reinvigorate internal resources to improve your situation or change your environment including moving on. This book distills current clinical papers and research; provides assessment tools and guidelines to pinpoint, avoid, and/or limit unnecessary distress and strengthen one's inner life. It also offers recommendations for further exploration on the topic. If nothing else, its goal is to raise awareness that secondary stress is a danger. The denial and avoidance of dealing with the immense stress present in modern health care are alarming. Professionals seem so discouraged at times that they do not even consider—given the culture and their own personal resources—that there are possible practical approaches to deal with environmental and intrapersonal sources of stress in health care settings. Instead, unfortunately, they just sleepwalk, march on, or march out.

In a session with a very competent professional who was starting to manifest early symptoms of chronic secondary stress such as hypersensitivity, increased daily use of alcohol, and sleep disturbance, the therapist asked how he would characterize his own problem. He said, "I may not be burned out yet." Then, after a brief pause, he smiled slightly and added, "But I think I'm experiencing at least a 'brown out!'" Acknowledging his insight, the therapist asked that given the precarious situation in which he recognized himself, what type of self-care protocol had he designed for himself and used to prevent further deterioration of his emotional well-being? In response, after sighing, he said, "I only wish I had the time for something like that!"

Time, of course, is especially precious for those in clinical practice. To keep afloat, they need to schedule their priorities and ensure that what is done is accomplished in the most effective way possible. And in this sorting process, oneself is often at the bottom of the priority list. *Overcoming Secondary Stress in Medical and Nursing Practice* is designed with these realities and practices in mind. Without a clear awareness of the challenges of professional health care and the simple, yet powerful, ways to remain a passionate, psychologically healthy physician, physician's assistant, or nurse and appreciate the need to strengthen one's "inner life," one's career may become derailed and one's personal life unduly suffer.

This book is presented in a way that fosters an appreciation of the essential elements of the problem of secondary stress. It will help you to answer the question, "Why am I feeling so stressed or so numb?" Most of these elements will be obvious; some may prove quite surprising. This book will suggest guidelines for the development of a personally designed self-care protocol as well as information on maintaining perspective, reframing perceptions, and increasing self-knowledge as a way of learning and benefiting from, rather than just being pulled down by, stressful encounters. The authors have reviewed major portions of the stress-related research and clinical papers published over the past 10 years. The bibliography in this volume is extensive and includes both classical and recent major works on the topic and websites that might be helpful, including links to online videos of prominent clinicians and researchers working on issues of secondary stress and burnout. Beyond what is written in the five chapters and epilogue, all sources provide helpful follow-up reading for those wishing to do so.

The brevity of the book is also intentional, because of our awareness of the time constraints of clinicians. The goal then is to provide a concise, practical, and engaging book that incorporates current clinical work and research that will be of specific interest to physicians, physician assistants, and nurses who are committed to caring for others while caring for self. In short, this clinical guide is written primarily for those *psychologically healthy* clinicians who want to understand, avoid, and limit, as much as is possible, the secondary stress in their own lives and at the same time remain passionate about their work.

Direct care providers realize that "for every poisoned worker there are a dozen with sub-clinical toxicity."[9] Using this as a metaphor for secondary stress, for every case of serious impairment, there are many nurses, physician assistants, and physicians who are beginning to manifest symptoms of chronic or acute secondary stress but may not even realize it until well after the fact and until well after they have made a decision to exit their current position or the profession. Consider the experience of a graduate nursing student who confided to her nursing instructor.

In a surprise phone call, three weeks before the end of the term, the nursing professor learned that one of her most outstanding graduate nursing students had decided to leave nursing. The instructor shared her surprise with the student but did not directly discourage her. Instead, she asked the student to share her reasons for this decision and her plans going forward. The student described her work environment, a fast-paced, clinical unit where she had hardly any time to spend with patients and families and where the nurse manager was more like an unforgiving "drill sergeant" barking orders and publicly calling out the staff. Most staff worked in fear and silence, but the stress was taking its toll—lack of sleep, ruminating thoughts, and hypersensitivity. "The only thing that has been holding me back is my tuition reimbursement benefit, but my decision is made, I am resigning and opening my own business." The instructor listened supportively and encouraged the student to postpone her exit at least until she finished her coursework for this term. The student agreed to this plan, and the instructor gave the student the name of a counselor who might help her sort out her "options" in nursing or otherwise. "And if after careful consideration you decide to pursue that business," the instructor offered, "let me know and I will be one of your first customers."

As the academic year progressed, the instructor often thought of this student wondering if she had been lost to the nursing profession. Shortly before the end of the next academic year, there was another call from student to instructor. "I will see you at graduation," the student exclaimed, "and I hope you will be there. I got into counseling and looked at my options. I have a new nursing position taking care of breast cancer patients. The staff and the setting are great. I cannot wait to get to work every day and I am so happy I made the decision to stay in nursing."

This story highlights the need for a clinically sound book that can be useful in helping health professionals and everyone in a field in which significant impairment is a constant possibility when care is not taken to understand, to carefully confront and prevent personal and systemic sources of secondary stress. To reiterate, the most insidious danger to physicians, physician assistants, and nurses is *denial*. Fortunately, this factor atrophies of its own accord once we accept the following simple reality: *The seeds of secondary stress and the seeds of true passionate involvement in the fields of medicine and nursing are actually the same seeds.*

The question is not *whether* stress will appear and take a toll on those working in health care; it is rather to what extent professionals take essential steps to appreciate, minimize, and learn from this stress to continue—and even deepen—their roles as helpers and healers. Understanding stress unique to health care work and developing a personal self-care protocol can help immeasurably in this regard, and that is what *Overcoming Secondary Stress in Medical and Nursing Practice* is designed to encourage.

To foster this understanding and concomitant action, the chapters of this book are as follows. Chapter 1 ("Tacking on Dangerous Psychological Waters: Appreciating the Factors Involved in Chronic and Acute Secondary Stress") includes models of chronic secondary stress (often referred to as *burnout, compassion fatigue,* or *moral distress*) and its acute counterpart, vicarious posttraumatic stress. Chapter 1 identifies behaviors and tools to increase awareness of bodily and cognitive responses to stressors and to differentiate between reactions and planned responses in stressful situations. It also focuses on the role that toxic parts of the health care system, including clinical environments, play in exacerbating personal stress and on the role of the individual in contributing to healthy work environments.

Chapter 2 ("Wicked Problems in Health Care: Identifying, Reframing, Sufficing, and Forgiving Oneself") is new to this edition and explores the concept of "wicked problems" as contrasted with "tame problems" in the health care environment. Wicked problems are never-ending, morphing problems that serve as a major source of secondary stress for physicians, physician assistants, and nurses. This chapter also features a new section Guilt and Facing the Coronavirus: A Guide for Professional Helpers and Healers Experiencing Traumatic Countertransference by Robert Wicks.

Chapter 3 ("'Riding the Dragon': Enhancing Self-Knowledge and Self-Talk in the Health Care Professional") distills essential information on approaches to increasing self-awareness by summarizing findings on increasing emotional resilience that is available in a variety of literatures and databases including psychology, psychiatry, medicine, physician assistant, and nursing. Chapter 3 emphasizes the importance of reflection and developing perspective as well as how professional stereotypes can interfere in effective communication often fueling conflict in professional practice roles. Included also is an exploration of the relationship between anger and health; the concept of stupidity and moving beyond it; the role of humor in health, healing, and the creation of healthy work environments. Chapter 3 also offers a specially designed Medical/ Nursing Professional Secondary Stress Self-Awareness Questionnaire, which assists readers in creating their own profile with respect to vulnerability, strength, and the pressures of life in clinical fields. By using it alone, with a mentor, or in a small group, it can aid in providing information that will enhance self-awareness and stress prevention.

Chapter 4 ("Drawing from the Well of Wisdom: Three Core Spiritual Approaches to Maintaining Perspective and Strengthening the Inner Life of Medical and Nursing Professionals") explores the intertwined roles of mind, body, and spirit and how core spiritual wisdom from a world religion perspective—and the applied psychology that evolves from this—can be used in one's life as a way of developing and maintaining perspective, balance, and a renewed sense of meaning. This chapter distills the core of some of Wicks's writing on these topics in past decades with an eye to what would be practical and essential for those practicing medicine and nursing—whether they are religious or not—to consider, given the intensity of their work, the richness of their lives and their sense of mission with regard to caring. Chapter 4 also includes a review of meditative techniques, how to listen to others, and how to combat perfectionistic tendencies. A realistic exploration of work–life balance is also included and contrasted with body–mind–spirit balance, which can contribute to work–life balance.

Chapter 5 ("The Simple Care of a Hopeful Heart: Developing a Personally Designed Self-Care Protocol") builds on and evolves from the previous four chapters. It explores the concepts of happiness and career satisfaction, self-respect, and the ability to discern the differences between toxic and healthy work environments. It presents practical guidelines on developing a personally designed self-care protocol to decrease vulnerability to the natural pressures of being a professional in the health care setting. As in preceding chapters, there are exercises that can be completed to improve self-awareness as a systematic way to enhance one's approach to self-care and to strengthening one's inner life.

Finally, as the brief epilogue's title ("Passionate Journeys: Returning to the Wonders of Medical and Nursing Practice") indicates, this book is also about rekindling the passion that led to a professional role in the healing arts. A caution—pondering some of these recommended time-consuming stress-reduction steps may seem stressful! On the other hand, denying the dangers posed by secondary stress and resisting a reasonable process of self-knowledge and self-care under the guise that it too is impractical must be circumvented. Given this contrasting view, the premise of this book is tied to a significantly different question: Who in their right mind would not take the time to ponder the *essentials* of self-knowledge, self-care, and secondary stress?

Everything that initially attracted people to these fascinating, meaningful, and rewarding professions are still present in some form. However, care must be taken to preserve and enhance a sense of personal and professional well-being and perspective so that the passion for caring and healing is not lost. By using knowledge and humility (the two key elements of wisdom) when faced with the stress of the work, one's passion and commitment can deepen and mature. The goal of this brief work is based squarely on this belief and hope.

Recommended Material

It is not always possible to hear and see one of the authors of the book that you are reading. Robert Wicks's brief talks on the following subjects can be found on YouTube at the following sites. These talks can provide some direction for your own work on overcoming secondary stress.

On Living Authentically https://www.youtube.com/watch?v= Db9VW_JeoLk

On Dealing With Failure https://www.youtube.com/watch?v= KLGRNJU0BF4

References

1. DevOps Enterprise Summit. Christina Maslach: Understanding job burnout. https://itrevolution.com/understanding-job-burnout-christina-maslach/ Published February 2019. Accessed April 29, 2020.

2. American Medical Association. Stepsforward: burnout and well being modules. https://edhub.ama-assn.org/steps-forward/module/2702510. Published 2020. Accessed April 29, 2020.

3. Accreditation Review Commission on Education for the Physician Assistant, Inc. *Accreditation Standards for Physician Assistant Education.* 5th ed. Johns Creek, GA: ARC:PA; 2020.

4. American Nurses Association. Healthy work environment. https://www.nursingworld.org/practice-policy/work-environment/. Accessed April 29, 2020.

5. Peckham C. Physician burnout: it just keeps getting worse. https://www.medscape.com/viewarticle/838437_1. Published April 30, 2015, April 30. Accessed February 29, 2020.

6. Eiser A. *The Ethos of Medicine in Post Modern America.* Lanham, MD: Lexington Books; 2014.

7. Coplan B, McCall TC, Smith M, Gellert VL, Essary AC. Burnout, job satisfaction and stress levels of physician assistants. *Journal of the American Academy of Physician Assistants.* 2018;31(9):42–46.

8. Carpenter H. American Nurses Association health risk appraisal: Three years later. *American Nurse Today.* Pp. 1–43 https://www.cdc.gov/niosh/topics/workschedules/pdfs/CARPENTER_ANAfinal-Presentation.pdf. Published January 2017. Accessed February 29, 2020.

9. Block D. Foreword. In: Scott CD, Hawk J, eds., *Heal thyself: The health of healthcare professionals.* New York, NY: Brunner Mazel; 1986: 1–13.

Tacking on Dangerous Psychological Waters

Appreciating the Factors Involved in Chronic and Acute Secondary Stress

Objectives

- Define models of stress including primary and secondary stress, burnout and compassion fatigue, and posttraumatic stress syndrome (PTSD).
- Identify signs, symptoms, and levels of burnout.
- Review the impact of work culture on stress and burnout.
- Explore the importance of self-awareness and thought patterns in determining responses to stress.
- Review the meaning of vicarious PTSD and how it manifests in clinical practice.
- Review strategies to self-debrief and to assist others to debrief stressful situations.
- Identify the potential of COVID-19 experiences to enhance self-awareness and self-care.
- Identify ways to contribute to healthy work environments as colleague or leader/manager.

When you come to the end of your rope, tie a knot and hang on.
—Franklin Delano Roosevelt

Kylie was accepted into a Physician Assistant Program after earning a biomedical engineering degree and working 5 years in the health IT industry. She had experienced a serious health problem and was inspired by a physician assistant (PA) who was especially instrumental in her care and recovery. Emergency medicine was her first love, and 1 year after graduation, she secured a position in an inner-city emergency department (ED) where she has practiced for the last 5 years. Weeks of 12-hour shifts caring for critically ill COVID-19 patients had pushed Kylie to the brink. "I am exhausted, depressed and I do not feel safe. I can't even visit my Mom who has dementia for fear of infecting her. I tried to talk to the ED director who is usually so understanding, but she brushed me off, 'This is what we signed on for so stop complaining and go with the flow!"—difficult to do when the flow is a tsunami. Like many health professionals working in modern health care, Kylie is reconsidering her career choice.

Secondary stress represents the stress caused by the pressures placed on professionals who care for others in need. To understand the causes, symptoms, and prevention/mitigation interventions, it is helpful to break down secondary stress into three components:

- Chronic secondary stress—also known as burnout, compassion fatigue, or moral distress.
- Acute secondary stress—sometimes referred to as secondary traumatic stress and vicarious PTSD.
- Unique unhealthy aspects of the contemporary health care culture.

One of the earliest researchers of the human stress response, Hans Selye, described the general adaptation syndrome in which the body responds to stress of any kind with a unified defense mechanism. This reaction to stress can raise the body's resistance to stressful agents both physical and psychological and can also be used to protect against illness. However, when the reaction is faulty or overly prolonged, it can also produce disease and even death.[1] An exploration of the components of stress highlights the many systemic stressors in medicine and nursing that must be faced as well as the inner resources and personal growing edges that will emerge in the process of meeting them.

Facing stressful obstacles is like tacking through rough waters. In his book *First You Have to Row a Little Boat*, Richard Bode describes this approach quite well:

To tack a boat, to sail a zigzag course, is not to deny our destination or our destiny—despite how it may appear to those who never dare to take the tiller in their hand. Just the opposite: It's to recognize the obstacles that stand between ourselves and where we want to go, and then to maneuver with patience and fortitude, making the most of each leg of our journey, until we reach our landfall.[2p49]

"Tacking" is an ideal metaphor for the way medical and nursing professionals must face pressures in general and chronic secondary stress in particular. To ignore what must be faced or to simply seek to take everything head on may be disastrous both personally and professionally. On the other hand, knowledge about the mechanisms of secondary stress and our unique responses to stressors may help us to psychologically tack the stressful waters so we can make the most of all that we face as caregivers.

Chronic Secondary Stress

Russian playwright Anton Chekhov once proclaimed, "Any idiot can face a crisis—it's this day-to-day living that wears you out." A 2006 study of Minnesota medical students reported a 45 percent rate of burnout including emotional exhaustion, depersonalization, and a low sense of personal accomplishment. The study results also revealed that in addition to work related events, negative personal life events also correlated highly with the risk of burnout.[3]

Eiser[4] asserts that physician depersonalization is associated with worse patient outcomes. "Burnout begets lower patient satisfaction as the physician also experiences dissatisfaction" (Eiser AR, Ibid., p. 135). He attributes this phenomenon to the decline of physician status in society, where physicians "were expected to make great personal sacrifice, but also . . . occupied a position that was honored and rewarded both financially and emotionally" (Eiser AR, Op.Cit., p. 135). In concert with Eiser's[4] views, Clever, also a physician, aptly notes, "We cannot relieve the suffering of others if we, ourselves, are suffering."[5,6p393] Such unfortunate suffering can occur slowly, quietly, almost imperceptibly.

Burnout is also reported in studies of PAs and nurses. In a study of PAs, Coplan et al.[7] reported that PAs' experience modest levels of burnout. Study participants reported spending too many hours at work and more female PAs than male PAs (32.2 percent vs. 25.6 percent) have left a position because of stress.

The American Nurses Association conducted a health risk appraisal of 13,500 registered nurses between 2013 and 2016.[8] This study, which has served as the impetus for the American Nurses Association's Healthy Work Environment initiative, revealed that 82 percent of responding nurses cited workplace stress as a health risk. The culture of health care has evolved into a crucible of stress for all health professionals who are committed to caring for others but who need also to care for themselves.

In the novel *The Case of Lucy Bending*, the psychiatrist laments in a way that rings all too true for medical and nursing professionals in real life:

> Most laymen, he supposed, believed psychiatrists fell apart under the weight of other people's problems. Dr. Theodore Levin had another theory. He feared that a psychiatrist's life force gradually leaked out. It was expended on sympathy, understanding, and the obsessive need to heal and help create whole lives. Other people's lives. But always from the outside. Always the observer. Then one day he would wake up and discover that he himself was empty, drained.[9p42]

An Insidious Unnecessarily Unhealthy Culture

Communications theorist Marshall McLuhan once posed the following question: "If the temperature of the bath rises one degree every ten minutes, how will the bather know when to scream?" In no setting is this question a more apt one to consider than in health care settings that contribute to the unhealthy lifestyles of their staffs—oft times under the guise of requirements for good patient care. Summers and Summers's recent book *Saving Lives: Why the Media's Portrayal of Nursing Puts Us All at Risk* is a stark reminder of how the media reinforces myths and stereotypes of nurses. They point to the international nursing shortage as a symptom of how the nursing profession is generally portrayed as

> a critical factor underlying the shortage is the huge gap between the actual nature and value of nursing, on the one hand, and what policy makers, career seekers, and the public at large *believe* about nursing on the other. Nursing has not received adequate resources because it continues to be seen as a peripheral, menial job for women with few other options. Legislative reforms and better funding will not be enough,

vital as those steps are. All the numbers measuring the short-age reflect what starts in our minds. The shortage cannot be resolved until public understanding improves. We must change how the world *thinks* about nursing.[10p20]

The news media's portrayal of nurses during the recent COVID-19 pandemic may generate a more realistic image of nurses, their extensive knowledge base, and their deep practice skills, given the media's characterization of "nurses as heroes." This positive portrayal also extends to all other medical practitioners, particularly first responders and those who staff emergency departments and intensive care units. On the other hand, the recent pandemic has created unprecedented stress for medical and nursing professionals who risked their health to care for others in environments ill prepared for the task with respect to the availability of personal protective equipment, testing, treatments, and hospital capacity. It is a historical fact that societies learn from pandemics, improving infrastructure and intervention as a function of lessons learned. Will the lessons of COVID-19 extend to improving clinical environments and ameliorating the stress of medical and nursing professionals, the health care system's most precious commodities? Or will the pandemic experiences of medical and nursing professionals discourage others from seeking health professional careers?

During a grand rounds on the topic of medical practice and secondary stress, we discussed the important balance that needs to be met. On the one hand, contemporary medicine is intense—long hours, poor staffing, life and death decisions, lengthy documentation requirements, and relationships with staff and patients all take their toll. On the other hand, there are elements in health care that have crept quietly into the culture that can be applied individually or systemically in ways that lessen unnecessary stress. For example, policies can be enacted to prevent workaholism, sleep deprivation, and other stressors of training instead of viewing them as part and parcel of the practice scene. If this is not done, the problem just perpetuates itself. As one practicing physician, who was interviewed for a study on residents in family medicine, said about the carryover of the time pressures he experienced in training, "You may be able to get out of the residency, but it's real hard to get the residency out of you." Careful examination of this situation though can lead to other, more hopeful conclusions. These points and a myriad of other factors make it imperative that we have a greater understanding of chronic secondary stress (burnout, compassion fatigue) if self-understanding and care are to be based on sound awareness of the challenges and dangers present in health care.

Definition and Causes of Burnout

Edelwich and Brodsky, in one of the first academic book-length treatments of the topic of burnout, defined it as a "progressive loss of idealism, energy, and purpose experienced by people in the helping professions."[11p14] Freudenberger, who coined the term *burnout*, described it as "a depletion or exhaustion of a person's mental and physical resources attributed to his or her prolonged, yet unsuccessful striving toward unrealistic expectations, internally or externally derived."[12p223] Since Freudenberger introduced this term, the concept of burnout has been questioned as to its necessity because the same symptoms and signs are seen in other disorders (depression, anxiety). However, many in the field, believe that the term is still quite helpful in highlighting and validating the extremes of stress that can be experienced by medical and nursing professionals. Moreover, the term *burnout* represents a comprehensive way to look at the emotional stress that health care workers uniquely experience in their work. The United Nations Policy Brief on COVID-19 and the Need for Action on Mental Health each point to the immediate need for services for frontline clinical workers in the COVID-19 pandemic.

> First responders and frontline workers, particularly workers in health and long-term care play a crucial role in fighting the outbreak and saving lives. However, they are under exceptional stress, being faced with extreme workloads, difficult decisions, risks of becoming infected and spreading infection to families and communities and witnessing deaths of patients. Stigmatization of these workers is common in too many communities. There have been reports of suicide attempts and suicide death by health-care workers.[13p11]

The causes for burnout are legion. As Pfifferling helps us to appreciate, trying to pin down one source of impairment that health care professionals need to be aware of is futile: "As with diseases or conditions that do not have a single cause, there are multiple suggestions, as to the origin, contributing factors, and types of susceptible hosts."[14p3]

In an article on the topic of burnout, psychiatrist James Gill wryly notes that "helping people can be extremely hazardous to your physical and mental health."[15p21] His timeless description of who might be good candidates for burnout follows:

> Judging from the research done in recent years, along with clinical experience, it appears that those who fall into the following categories are generally the most vulnerable: (1) those who work exclusively with distressed persons; (2) those who work intensively with demanding people who feel entitled to assistance in solving their . . . problems; (3) those who are charged with the responsibility for too many individuals; (4) those who feel strongly motivated to work with people but who are prevented from doing so by too many administrative paperwork tasks; (5) those who have an inordinate need to save people from their undesirable situations but find the task impossible; (6) those who are very perfectionistic and thereby invite failure; (7) those who feel guilty about their own human needs (which, if met, would enable them to serve others with stamina, endurance and emotional equanimity); (8) those who are too idealistic in their aims; (9) those whose personality is such that they need to champion underdogs; (10) those who cannot tolerate variety, novelty, or diversion in their work life; and (11) those who lack criteria for measuring the success of their undertakings but who experience an intense need to know that they are doing a good job.[15p21]

Most researchers and authors on the topic of burnout have developed their own tailored list of the causes of burnout (Box 1.1), but

> there is much overlap, and all seem to point to the problem as being a *lack* that produces frustration. It can be a deficiency— the lack of education, opportunity, free time, ability, chance to ventilate, institutional power, variety, meaningful tasks, criteria to measure impact, coping mechanisms, staff harmony, professional and personal recognition, insight into one's motivations, balance in one's schedule, and emotional distance from the client population. . . . And because these factors are present to

Box 1.1 Causes of Burnout

1. Inadequate quiet time—physical rest, cultural diversion, further education, and personal psychological replenishment
2. Vague criteria for success and/or inadequate positive feedback on efforts made
3. Guilt over failures and over taking out time to nurture oneself properly to deal with one's own legitimate needs
4. Unrealistic ideals that are threatening rather than generally motivating
5. Inability to deal with anger or other interpersonal tensions
6. Extreme need to be liked by others, prompting unrealistic involvement with others
7. Neglect of emotional, physical, and spiritual needs
8. Poor community life and/or unrealistic expectations and needs surrounding the support and love of others for us
9. Working with people (peers, superiors, those coming for help) who have burnout
10. Extreme powerlessness to effect needed change or being overwhelmed by paperwork and administrative tasks
11. Fear of providing feedback or questioning managers and colleagues
12. Serious lack of appreciation by our superiors, colleagues, or those whom we are trying to serve
13. Sexism, ageism, racism, or other prejudice experienced directly in our lives and work
14. High conflict in the family, home, work, or living environment
15. Serious lack of charity and kindness among those with whom we must live or work
16. Extreme change during times in life when maturational crises and adjustments are also occurring (e.g., a 48-year-old physician who is being asked to work with patients diagnosed with cancer at a time when she has just been diagnosed with cancer herself)

17. Seeing money wasted on projects that seem to have no relation to helping people or improving the health care system
18. Not having the freedom or power to deal with or absent oneself from regularly occurring stressful events
19. Failure to curb one's immature reasons for helping others and to develop more mature ones in the process
20. The "savior complex"—inability to recognize what we can and cannot do in helping others in need
21. Inability to say no to those who take advantage of your willingness to help.
22. Overstimulation or isolation and alienation

some degree in every human service setting, the potential for burnout is always present."[16p336]

Consequently, every healing professional is in danger of impairment in some way *to some extent*. Yet, care is provided in most settings only to those professionals who are so seriously impaired as to be required by their state boards to seek out help. Although programs for impaired medical and nursing professionals are essential, as in the case of physical problems or addictions, prevention or early treatment is obviously a preferable step to later intervention. However, as reported in the *Annals of Internal Medicine*,

> Self-care is not a part of the physician's professional training and typically is low on a physician's list of priorities. "Physicians deal with [other people's] problems all day, but they're the least likely to raise their own personal problems. They don't easily admit that they're under stress," remarked [neurologist T. Jock] Murray. Approximately one third of physicians do not have a doctor according to a study that examined graduates of the Johns Hopkins School of Medicine.[17p145]

This lack of attention by physicians to self-care can effect patient outcomes according to Halbesleben and Rothert's[18] study of 178 matched pairs of patients and the physicians who cared for them. The depersonalization dimension of physician burnout correlated with patients' lower satisfaction with their care and longer post discharge recovery times. Self-care should be a significant component of all health professional curricula.

In an earlier work on effective emotional management for physicians and their medical organizations, Sotile and Sotile cluster some of the research on physician stress under the theme of "betrayal."[19] To use their wording, "Remember: Stress that is highly demanding but also meaningful and controllable is healthy stress, not the sort that promotes burnout. Our counseling and consulting experience suggest that what *really* stresses physicians is feeling betrayed, or double-crossed."[19p336] What is meant by this "betrayal" is illustrated in a quote by a physician from a Canadian survey by Sullivan and Burke:

> I believe that most physicians unconsciously contracted with society to pursue their profession to the utmost of their ability and energy, to keep up their skills and do whatever was needed to promote patient care. In return, we expected respect, the equipment to do the job and freedom from financial anxieties. All 3 of these expectations have been abrogated, yet we continue to fulfill our side of the contract in confusion, disbelief and a sense of betrayal.[20p525]

Eiser resonates with this point of view asserting that

> physician morale globally is one of mutual distress. . . . The loss of status of the health professional reverberates through the clinical encounter and adversely affects patients as well as the physicians themselves. The social forces that wrought these changes include the extensive media coverage of medicine's fault, electronic communication, loss of community, moral relativism, consumerist ideology, corporate control of medical practice.[4p135]

Loss of autonomy and status engenders conflict within work relationships and at home. *Loss of autonomy* occurs you realize that you are no longer making decisions and choices based on what you value and identify as important and that your decisions are having less impact to the degree that you seem to have no control at all. Thus, work becomes less satisfying and meaningful. The advent of corporate health care and large, impersonal health systems, practice by protocol, and new insurer norms has resulted in physicians, PAs, and nurse practitioners experiencing a dramatic decrease in a sense of control. When the impact of this starts to psychologically "infect" a health care organization, it can set the stage for group burnout, because negativity is so emotionally contagious.

Changes in patient–physician relationships and *conflicts with peers, staff, and administration* are the other two areas on which Sotile and Sotile focus.[19] In relationships with patients, it is easy for health care professionals to identify with the stress that can arise from interactions with persons who relate in a difficult manner. There are classic styles that fit into this category (e.g., passive aggressive, overtly hostile, demanding especially with respect to time, etc.). One colleague recently quipped: "I really think there are only five difficult patients in the world and they just move from hospital to hospital." Eiser cites the postmodern organization, characterized by ambiguity, a flattening of traditional hierarchies and shifting power relationships, as a tsunami of stressors effecting medical and nursing professionals as well as hospital administrators.[4p139]

Sometimes a patient becomes difficult to deal with for a myriad of reasons (e.g., the health care professional is exhausted from being on call all night or completing a 12-hour shift), and this inadvertently exacerbates the situation. In one observation of interactions in a pediatric emergency department, the observer noted the different styles of workers and their effect on one patient. A 30-year-old woman brought in her youngest child, a 1½-year-old, who was having respiratory problems and a rising fever. When she first brought the child in at midnight, both the physician (who was struggling with English) and the nurse listened carefully to the problem, explained possible causes, and suggested several approaches. Once there was agreement on the approach, treatment was careful, kind, and swift. The mother of the patient reported great satisfaction with the treatment provided for her child and the information given to her.

When the woman had to revisit the same emergency department the next morning to clarify one of the forms of treatment and to request assistance with it, she encountered three physicians and a nurse when she entered the unit. She noted that not one of them stood to greet her or made eye contact. Instead, they remained focused on their tasks, writing notes and talking on the phone. As the mother explained her needs, they seemed confused and impervious as to how to meet them. As the woman became more fearful about whether her needs would be met, one of the physicians became more strident as to what she should do. When the woman expressed anger, rather than letting her vent and express understanding as to how she felt, the physician kept repeating to the child's mother, "*You* are not listening. *You* are not listening!" The physician in question did not seem to realize that the patient was not the only one having a problem listening. The physician was not perceiving the emotions masking the fear this mother was experiencing concerning her child. The situation could have been managed much differently before it became a stressful situation for both the patient and the physician. The overall lesson is that there is enough unavoidable stress in the health care setting without communicating to both patients and colleagues in a way that unnecessarily increases stress. When patients, particularly pediatric and geriatric patients, and their families, have increased stress due to poor physician/nurse-patient communications, it is the caregiver who ultimately is the recipient of the patient's ire. However, it is difficult for some medical and nursing professionals to develop a sufficiently sound level of self-awareness to discern the nuances of patient communication on every occasion. *However, increasing self-awareness is a self-care goal that should be seriously pursued.* Self-awareness leads to more effective self-regulation, the conscious planning or responses instead of automatic reactivity. (See the discussion in Chapter 3 on approaches to self-awareness.)

In terms of conflict with peers, staff, and administrators, Sotile and Sotile rely on a 1999 survey conducted for the American Academy of Physician Executives, which elicited types of conflicts experienced in health care environments.[19] Eiser also identifies types of conflict experienced by physicians in contemporary health care environments.[4] These sources and types of conflict are represented in Table 1.1.

The list in Table 1.1 is only part of the story. The danger of burnout, particularly in the context of the recent pandemic, remains a serious threat to the psychological welfare of health care professionals and those they serve. Therefore, a greater awareness of the form, causes, and manifestations of compassion fatigue or burnout is necessary. It should be noted that compassion fatigue is a type of burnout but with more rapid onset and resolution. The following statements by medical and nursing health professionals should be viewed as less a part of the territory of working in health care settings and more as symptoms of impending burnout that require vigilance.

Table 1.1 Sources and Types of Physician Conflict with Peers, Staff, and
Administrators

Peer Conflict	*Conflict With Administrators*
Schedules and calendars	Disagreement about values
Approaches to patient management	Lack of consistency in their actions
Sharing workload	Micromanagement
Clinic or laboratory space	Unfair treatment
Management of budget for a group/unit	Discrimination, gender and otherwise
Balancing patient care, teaching, and research	Salary negotiations
Authorship disputes	Broken promises
Failure to deal with their low performers	Clinical and other workload issues
	Ethical dilemmas
Conflict With Supervisees	*Conflict With System Changes*
Conflict among supervisees	Loss of autonomy and erosion of
Disparate expectations for performance	practice authority
Dealing with the low performer	Problems with insurance claims
Workloads and schedules	Corporate driven practice guidelines,
Inappropriate personal relationships at work	including order sets and protocols
Volume and quality of work	Public online patient ratings of
Unwillingness to change practice or behavior	physicians
Supervision outside the hierarchy	Computerization and
	hyper-information

Source: Sotile MW, Sotile MO, *The Resilient Physician* (Chicago: American Medical Association; 2002)—summarized from Aschenbrener CA, Siders CT, Managing low to -mid intensity conflict in the health care setting, *The Physician Executive*. 1999;25:44–50, and Eiser AR, *The Ethos of Medicine in Postmodern America* (Lanham MD: Lexington Books; 2014).

- *Cynicism*: "I just see this as a job, a paycheck. Health care is not what it used to be. Nothing is going to change. People ask me such trivial questions and burden me with stupid things."
- *Workaholism*: "I need to constantly check my email and phone mail even when I am not working on the weekend." "My husband and I need to earn a down payment for a house, so I have to work more shifts than I'd like."
- *Isolation*: "I really don't feel part of things on the unit. The other nurses (physicians, emergency medical services personnel, X-ray technicians, respiratory therapists, etc.) are nice people, but I feel so different and removed from them. I never discuss my work or personal life with any of them."
- *Boredom*: "I am so tired of doing the same thing every day. When I'm not killing myself, I'm bored to tears. If I hadn't invested so

much in this field already, I would get out. I can't wait until the end of a shift."

- *Depletion*: "I feel it is taking me longer and longer to do less and less. I no longer feel the passion about the job as I did in the past. I am tired before I begin. I don't quite dread going into work, but it certainly is getting to that point. All I think about is the job."
- *Conflict*: "Everything seems to get on my nerves now. I argue with the patients, am irritable with the staff, and am no fun to be with at home. I also resent having to deal with patients' families and feel that everyone is asking too much of me."
- *Arrogance*: "I wish I didn't have to deal with such incompetent co-workers. Also, I wish the patients would just do what I tell them and not ask so many questions. One even had the nerve to ask for a second opinion when I told her my diagnosis and treatment plan."
- *Helplessness*: "I am not sure I really can do anything to change my situation. This is the workload I must deal with, plain and simple. I know if I complain, I might be fired. Also, my sleeping is often disturbed, I have no time for family and friends, my sinuses are always bothering me, and I know I drink too much coffee in the morning and wine in the evening."

Rather than only avoiding the dangers of burnout (as good as this may be), professionals in health care should also take clear steps to prevent acceleration of stress that is endemic to practice in the fields of medicine and nursing. To do this, several steps can be taken:

1. Appreciate the levels of burnout and how they might apply to you.
2. Conduct frequent self-appraisals. Take time to identify potential problem areas and review how they are being addressed by developing a self-tailored *personality dysfunction profile*.
3. Be aware of constructive approaches managers can take to prevent or lessen secondary stress in the environment.

Levels of Burnout

The symptoms of chronic secondary stress include frustration, depression, apathy, helplessness, impatience, disengagement, emotional depletion, cynicism, hopelessness, a significant decline in one's professional

---

Box 1.2 Level 1—Daily Burnout: A Sampling of Key Signs and Symptoms

- Mentally fatigued at the end of the day
- Feeling unappreciated, frustrated, bored, tense, or angry as a result of a contact(s) with patients, colleagues, supervisors, superiors, assistants, or other potentially significant people
- Experiencing physical symptoms (e.g., headache, backache, upset stomach, etc.)
- Pace of day's activities and/or requirements of present tasks seem greater than personal or professional resources available
- Tasks required on job are repetitious, beyond the ability of the [caregiver], or require intensity on a continuous basis

Source: Wicks R, Parsons R, Capps D, Clinical Handbook of Pastoral Counselling. Vol. 3 (Mahwah, NJ: Paulist Press; 2003), used with permission.

---

self-esteem and confidence, feeling overwhelmed, and anhedonia. Despite the fact that the expression of burnout can be uniquely individual, it may be helpful to break down the possible progression of burnout recognizing that there is often overlap between the levels.

Gill described levels of burnout that could be most helpful to medical and nursing professionals.

The *first level* is characterized by signs and symptoms that are relatively mild, short in duration and occur only occasionally [see Box 1.2]. . . . The *second level* [see Box 1.3] is reached when signs and symptoms have become *more stable, last longer* and are *tougher* to get rid of. . . . The *third level* is experienced when signs and symptoms have become *chronic* and a *physical illness* has developed.[15p20] (emphasis added)

As explained elsewhere, this

commonsense breakdown (of the levels of burnout) is very much in line with the medical model and there is some overlap between levels of burnout. While they could be applied to any

Box 1.3 Level 2—Minor Stress Becomes Distress: Some
Major Signs and Symptoms

- Waning idealism and enthusiasm about being a [profes-
  sional caregiver]; disillusionment about [work] . . . surfac-
  ing on a regular basis
- Experiencing a general loss of interest in the . . . field for a
  period of a month or longer
- Pervasive feelings of boredom, stagnation, apathy, and
  frustration
- Unrealistic high expectations of self-perfectionism
- Taking on whatever the manager assigns—being the "go
  to" staff member, staying late at work
- Inability to "say no" to co-workers who have well devel-
  oped repertoires for avoiding work
- Being ruled by schedule; caring for more and more patients;
  being no longer attuned to them; viewing them imperson-
  ally and without thought
- Losing criteria with which to judge the effectiveness of
  work . . .
- Inability to get refreshed by the other elements in one's life
- Limiting contact with friends and family
- A loss of interest in professional resources (i.e., books, con-
  ferences, innovations, etc.) . . .
- Intermittent lengthy (week or more) periods of irritation,
  depression, and stress which do not seem to lift even with
  some effort to correct the apparent causes

Sources: Wicks R., Parsons R., Capps D, *Clinical Handbook of Pastoral Counselling.* Vol. 3
(Mahwah, NJ: Paulist Press, 2003), used with permission; Donnell GF, From the editor: you can't burnout unless you've been on fire! *Holistic Nursing Practice.* 2004;18(4):177.

physical or psychological constellation of symptoms and signs,
they provide a reasonable way of delineating a breakdown of
the burnout syndrome. The third level is self-explanatory. And
in line with what is known about serious prolonged countertransference [feelings on the helpers' part toward patients and

colleagues that have sources in their own past] . . . the signs, symptoms, and treatment are obvious. . . . If the [caregiver] is experiencing a life crisis and undergoing notable ongoing psychosomatic problems, then it means that preventive measures and self-administered treatments have failed. Psychological and medical assistance is necessary. This may mean entering or re-entering psychotherapy and obtaining, as advised by the therapist, medical help if necessary. Once this third level has been reached, burnout is severe, and remediation of the problem will likely take a good deal of time and effort.[16p337]

Preventative measures can be implemented before reaching Level 3 burnout. Because the seeds of burnout and the seeds of enthusiasm are the same seeds, anyone who truly cares can expect to ride the waves of burnout—and occasionally get knocked down by a rogue wave. Basic steps to take in averting burnout (Box 1.4) should, in most cases, prevent many of the difficulties. Level 1 burnout is experienced by all medical and nursing professionals at one time or another: boredom,

---

Box 1.4 Level 1—Daily Burnout: Steps for Dealing With "Daily Burnout"

1. Correcting one's cognitive errors so there is a greater recognition when we are exaggerating or personalizing situations in an inappropriate, negative way
2. Having a variety of activities in one's daily schedule
3. Getting sufficient rest
4. Faithfully incorporating some form of meditation [or quiet reflective time] into our daily schedule
5. Interacting on a regular basis with supportive friends
6. Being assertive
7. Getting proper nourishment and exercise
8. Being aware of the general principles set forth in the professional and self-help literature on stress management

Source: R Wicks R, Parsons R, Capps D, *Clinical Handbook of Pastoral Counselling.* Vol. 3 (Mahwah, NJ: Paulist Press; 2003), used with permission.

anger, minor physical problems, and periodic increases in the demands of work. Level 2 is

> where the burnout problem has become more severe and intractable to brief interventions, a more profound effort is necessary. [See Box 1.3.] Central to such actions is a willingness to reorient priorities and take risks with one's style of dealing with the world, which for some reason is not working optimally. To accomplish this, frequently one's colleagues . . . [and] mentor need to become involved. Their support and insight for dealing with the distress being felt is needed. The uncomfortable steps taken to unlock oneself from social problems and the temptation to deal with them in a single unproductive way (repetition compulsion) requires all the guidance and support one can obtain. In many cases, this also requires a break from work for a vacation or retreat, in order to distance oneself from the work for a time so that revitalization and reorientation can occur.[16p338]

Most medical and nursing professionals experience Level 1 burnout in the course of practicing. It is part of the ups and downs of being in an intense profession. Most health care professionals also experience Level 2 burnout at times, and some, unfortunately, Level 3. This is why awareness of the ever-present challenges of stress, being as self-aware as possible, using this self-knowledge (see Chapter 3 of this volume), developing a self-care protocol (see Chapter 5 of this volume), and knowing what both psychology and spirituality from the perspective of the world's religions have to offer all of us—whether we are religious or not—as a way of strengthening one's inner life (see Chapter 4 of this volume) are all essential. Beyond this, if we face stress wisely, not only do we lessen the chances of it turning into extreme distress; we also are able to learn from it in a way that deepens us. However, this requires both the right type of knowledge and the humility to turn to others for help when we do not progress as we should—not an easy task when people in the health care setting often transfer onto us the sense that we are omnipotent, always strong, and usually right.

The reality, however, is far from the projections that are put onto us. We all have personalities-in-process and growing edges. We are vulnerable to certain stressors, situations, and patient/colleague personality types who may unconsciously remind us of past negative interactions—a scolding parent, a school bully, or a critical teacher. As a result, it would help immeasurably to heighten our awareness, through self-questioning, of the sources of these vulnerable points so that we can act in our own behalf.

Personality Dysfunction Profile

Knowing what types of people and problems give you difficulty is the first step toward avoiding psychological vulnerability. For example, we develop negative impressions of people we meet for the first time, or we may have a chronic negative relationship with a colleague despite efforts on both sides. These situations could be the result of a *transference process*, a term used to describe the feelings that patients and therapists experience during psychotherapy. Transference usually refers to feelings that patients have for therapists that are rooted in relationships with significant others in the past (i.e., parents). Countertransference refers to feelings that therapists or clinical professionals have for patients, also rooted in past relationships in the therapist's family or life. Transference processes also occur in everyday life and may be the source of difficulties with patients, families, staff, or managers. Since these transference processes occur so frequently, we might refer to them humorously as "over the countertransference processes." For example, taking an instant dislike to a new staff member or feeling repulsed by a patient may be the outcome of transference processes, common occurrences in the course of a day. Given this, the following questions may provide an avenue to helpful information and insight concerning individual stress points. Ask yourself:

- What type of person "gets to you"?
- How do you deal with demanding patients?
- When young patients have a poor prognosis, what impact does this have on you?
- How do you blunt ("medicate") the pain you experience in clinical practice?
- In what instances do you "dump" on co-workers or subordinates?
- How do you handle unrealistic expectations of the medical/nursing staff and patients?

- What failures in the past haunt you now, and how have you learned from them?
- What procedures do you use to contain patients who direct their anger at the staff and stir up other patients and family members?
- What prevents you from fully responding to life as a person and as a medical or nursing professional?
- How do you handle unscheduled events in the day, such as multiple emergency admissions, equipment breakdowns or staff illness?
- What are the things that you lie to yourself about or hide from co-workers, patients, and family?
- What situations most easily trigger your anger?
- About what are you most insecure?
- What is having the greatest negative impact on both your professional and personal life?
- How have you addressed the imbalances in your home/work life (with spouse, children, friends, etc.) given the intensity of medical/nursing practice?
- How do you address problems in your department, such as under-staffing/poor staffing, ineffective management, incompetence/poor work ethic, chronic complaining, peer to peer bullying, rigidity, narrow compartmentalizing of responsibilities and not stepping beyond these roles, and overcompensating by some to deal with the weaknesses of others?
- Do you find yourself not listening to family or friends because you feel emotionally exhausted or because you feel that their problems are not as important as those of your patients?
- What themes run through your daydreams and night dreams?
- What recent cases or work situations produced in you the most guilt, resentment, or embarrassment?
- When and how often are you the most bored with work, and what do you do about it?
- What are the coping mechanisms you use when you feel over-whelmed? Withdrawal, isolation, lashing out, crying?

By periodically addressing questions like these fully and honestly, you will begin to see the areas where you have progressed and developed effective coping skills. Other areas will need attention—sometimes *constant* attention—given our ingrained personality styles. To ignore these areas is to court unnecessary stress. Even when you do not consciously feel the stress, this can translate into a problem. As one professional remarked when questioned about his problems with stress, "I don't think I really am usually under stress, but I think I'm a carrier!" When we do induce stress in others, there is often a cascade effect—they make life difficult for other workers, for family members, and so on, and this creates burnout contagion, which will eventually come back to haunt the "carrier" and decrease effectiveness in the organization. This situation requires that we have some familiarity with approaches to lessen the stress in those around us.

Constructive Approaches for Clinical Managers to Prevent or Lessen Chronic Secondary Stress

There are simple and direct approaches that can be used both in the work organization/unit and in one's personal life to decrease the severity of chronic secondary stress (burnout). The following are sample steps to consider, especially if you are a clinical manager or are in some form of supervisory role.

- Listen to the staff; solicit their opinions and provide opportunity for the venting of complaints. Create a regular meeting venue during which staff are encouraged to express their positive and negative observations and opinions.
- Keep the staff informed of policy and other changes that could affect their work situation.
- Know the difference between assertive, non-assertive, and aggressive behavior. Assertive behavior expresses thoughts and feelings from an "I" perspective, nonassertive behavior is withdrawing, isolating and holding back responses out of fear and anxiety and aggressive behavior attacks the other, using "You" messages that may accuse, blame, demean, or humiliate.
- Give "problem patients" some time to vent. Isolate problem patients from the earshot of other patients until matters can be resolved.
- Tell staff when they are doing a good job, when patients and families have given positive feedback. Publicly compliment staff on their good work and let physicians know when staff has been particularly helpful to their patients.

- Consider options when facing difficult situations. The same automatic response will often produce more difficulty. There are always options.
- Provide communication to staff of attempts made by administrators to improve the work environment so they realize their critiques are being addressed whenever possible.
- Treat the staff to lunch occasionally or stock the break room.
- Use humor when appropriate to lighten situations. Humor can connect you to others and heal relationships.
- Encourage creative problem-solving within staff's sphere of responsibility to encourage initiative and avoid the morale-destroying impact of micromanagement.
- Do not over rely on staff who are always willing to step to the plate. Intervene when you see staff taking advantage of "chronic helpers."
- Avoid catastrophizing, projecting the worst-case outcomes to every situation. Even when emotions are running high, at least try to stay calm and sound rational

The previously listed steps are only a sampling of simple approaches that one can use. They are offered to stimulate your creativity in this area. The important thing is to heighten awareness of the approaches you are already using that work well. In addition, employing these strategies will broaden your repertoire in the effort to lessen the possibility of chronic secondary stress in staff and work colleagues. Preventing burnout is a collective responsibility—not just the individual's. It is incumbent on medical and nursing professionals to be mindful of shared stressors and work together to create more balanced and healthier work environments.

Health care settings can be psychologically toxic. Throughout the months of the COVID-19 pandemic, stories and images flooded the media with descriptions of the toxic situations listed here:

- Hospital overcrowding creating work overload.
- Equipment shortages for both patients (i.e., ventilators) and staff (i.e., personal protective equipment).
- Fear of contagion and lack of testing (i.e., a survey of 27,000 nurses revealed that 84 percent had not been tested for COVID-19).[21.]
- Isolation and social distancing protocols that kept medical and nursing professionals from home and family.

- Revised visiting rules that prohibited family members from seeing patients even when death was imminent. One nurse held her video phone next to a dying patient so that the family could say "goodbye."
- Compromised financial resources from lack of reimbursement for elective procedures and the suspension of regular hospital admissions.
- Strain on and dissolution of medical practices.
- Post-COVID-19 hospital system layoffs and furloughs of clinical and support staff.

In a 2018 comprehensive review of the literature, West et al.[22] reported factors that contribute to burnout among physicians practicing in today's health care systems. Work factors include

- inefficient work processes particularly increased clinical burden such as computerized order entry.
- long work hours including excessive on call duties.
- excessive time on activities that are not personally meaningful.
- work–home conflicts.
- working in certain specialties such as emergency medicine, general internal medicine, and neurology.
- managing a private practice.

Organizational factors include

- lack of control over work environment.
- difficult relationships with leaders and senior administrators.

Individual factors include

- being a female physician.
- having children under 21.
- having a non-physician spouse.

In the American Nurses Association health risk appraisal survey of 13,500 nurses from 2013 to 2016,[23] nurse respondents identified the following factors as increasing stress levels in the work environment:

- 82 percent reported a significant level of workplace stress.
- 50 percent reported having been bullied at work, primarily by colleagues.

- 59 percent worked 10 hours or longer beyond the requirements of the shift.
- 57 percent reported a pattern of arriving to work early, staying late, and not taking breaks.
- 25 percent reported being physically assaulted by a patient or a patient's family member.
- 9 percent reported a concern for their physical safety at work.
- 45 percent identified the repositioning of heavy objects (i.e., patients) as risky even though 73 percent had access to technology to enhance safety
- 51 percent experienced musculoskeletal pain at work.
- 33 percent reported having workloads beyond their levels of comfort.

Finally, the Academy of Physician Assistants conducted a comprehensive survey of its members on burnout, job satisfaction, and stress levels. Coplan et al.[7] analyzed responses from 15,999 respondents, 16.5 percent of all U.S. PAs. While respondents overall reported "modest levels of burnout" and "are happy at work," they also listed the following stressors in their work environments.

- Feeling like a cog in a wheel.
- Low professional fulfillment.
- Excessive bureaucratic tasks including the increasing computerization of practice.
- Too many hours at work.
- Insufficient income.
- Inability to provide the level of quality care that patients need.
- Difficult patients.
- Difficult staff colleagues and employers.

These and other findings underpin the decision of the Accreditation Review Commission on Education for the Physician Assistant to include a new criterion in the Accreditation Standards for PA Education, that addresses the need to focus on the health and personal wellness of the PA. The new standard, B2.20 is "The curriculum must include instruction about provider personal wellness including the prevention of a) impairment and, b) burnout."[24]

The promotion of personal health and wellness and healthier work environments by physician, physician assistant and nursing groups will become even more important post pandemic. Pandemics throughout history have had a way of exposing the deficiencies of health systems and care environments. Finding ways for organizations and professionals themselves to mediate stressful environments and maintain health is the best way to prepare for the next major health disruption. Anything that can be done to deal with these sources of stress must be done. We realize this even more clearly when we recognize that in addition to chronic stress, there is an acute counterpart with which we must be familiar, Level 3 or acute secondary stress.

Acute Secondary Stress: Vicarious Posttraumatic Stress Disorder

Psychologist Jeffrey Kottler aptly described threats to his personal sense of well-being that were a byproduct of his work: "Never mind that we catch [our patients'] colds and flus, what about their pessimism, negativity. . . . Words creep back to haunt us. Those silent screams remain deafening."[25p8] What he is referencing here is the destabilization of one's own personality because of constant treatment of the severe psychological and physical trauma experienced by others.

Vicarious posttraumatic stress is a great danger today in health care settings. Not only must medical and nursing professionals deal with medical emergencies, they also must increasingly ease the suffering that patients experience due to the psychic trauma arising from abuse, rape and other physical assaults, terrorism, and, most recently, pandemic. When patients' suffering combines with the stress that health care professionals experience in their lives—including marital, financial, personal, and world instability—the result is quite psychologically toxic. Unrecognized or ignored, it could lead to severe impairment or a psychological "grayness" in how one experiences life, as well as a resultant inadequate treatment of patients as a function of one's emotional state.

One of the most sensible approaches to recognizing, limiting, avoiding, and even learning from the onset of vicarious PTSD is to conduct daily debriefings with yourself. A second approach is to have an organized way to question yourself to uncover the presence and/or duration of clusters of PTSD signs and symptoms. These two approaches go hand in hand. Wicks' personal account of this self-questioning process is strikingly useful today for medical and nursing professionals who are living through the disruptions of health care including a pandemic and its aftermath.

> Persons in the helping professions . . . at times lose distance and are temporarily swept away by the expectations, needs, painful experiences, and negativity of others. More than most people, they are confronted with negativity and sadness. Yet, they are educated to pick up these signs as early as possible, so they are not unnecessarily dragged down. We can learn much from how they avoid losing perspective or regain it when they temporarily lose their way. The distance they value can help us deal with the pain of others.
>
> There is much to remembering the Russian proverb: "When you live next to the cemetery, you can't cry for everyone who dies." Most of us, whether we are professional helpers or not, tend to personalize too much. We absorb the sadness, anxiety, and negativity of those around us. Sometimes we even feel this is expected of us. . . . As we listen to stories of terrible things that happen [or observe them] . . . we catch some of their futility, fear, vulnerability, and hopelessness rather than experiencing mere frustration or concern. We learn that no matter how professionally prepared we are, we are not immune to the psychological and spiritual dangers that arise in living a full life of involvement with others. I remember learning this the hard way myself.
>
> In 1994 I did a psychological debriefing of some of the relief workers evacuated from Rwanda's bloody civil war. I interviewed each person and gave them an opportunity to tell their stories. As they related the horrors they had experienced, they seemed to be grateful for an opportunity to vent. They recounted the details again and again, relating their feelings as well as descriptions of the events which triggered them. Their sense of futility, their feelings of guilt, their sense of alienation, their experiences with emotional outbursts, all came to the fore.
>
> In addition to listening, I gave them handouts on what to possibly expect down the road (problems sleeping, difficulties trusting and relating to others, flashbacks and the like). As I moved through the process of debriefing and providing

information so they could have a frame of reference for understanding their experiences, I thought to myself, "This is going pretty well." Then, something happened that shifted my whole experience.

During one of the final interviews, one of the relief workers related stories of how certain members of the Hutu tribe raped and dismembered their Tutsi foes. Soon, I noticed I was holding onto my chair for dear life. I was doing what some young people call "white knuckling it."

After the session, I did what I usually do after an intense encounter . . . a countertransferential review. (If time doesn't permit then, I do it at the end of the day—every day.) In doing this, I get in touch with my feelings by asking myself: What made me sad? Overwhelmed me? Sexually aroused me? Made me extremely happy or even confused me? Being brutally honest with myself, I try to put my finger on the pulse of my emotions.

The first thing that struck me about this particular session was the tight grip I had on the chair as the session with the relief worker progressed. "What was I feeling when I did this? Why did I do this?"

It didn't take me long to realize that their terrible stories had broken through my defenses and normal sense of distance and detachment. I was holding onto the chair because quite simply, I was frightened to death that if I didn't, I would be pulled into the vortex of darkness myself.

That recognition alone helped lessen the pain and my fearful uneasiness. I then proceeded with a . . . countertransferential review . . . used by therapists . . . to prevent the slide into unnecessary darkness and to learn—and thus benefit—from the events for the day.[26pp54-109]

The questions we can ask ourselves to determine whether vicarious PTSD may well be present are listed in (Box 1.5). (The guidelines of the profile for this syndrome noted in the American Psychiatric Association's *Diagnostic and Statistical Manual of Mental Disorders*, fifth edition, provide additional assistance as to what may constitute a significant problem in this area. It should be noted that PTSD is now included in a new category, Trauma and Stressor Related Disorders.

Box 1.5 Questions to Uncover Vicarious PTSD

If one or more of the following symptoms or signs have lasted longer than 1 month and are presently interfering in your personal and professional life, care must be taken to consider that the result of being constantly exposed to persons who have experienced trauma may be having a vicarious impact on the health care provider:

1. Do you find that you are re-experiencing past traumatic events via any of the following?
   a. Nightmares
   b. Intrusive thoughts
   c. Flashbacks to events
   d. Reliving events
   e. Association of events in present with past trauma or the traumatic experiences of others
2. Are you experiencing a blunting of affect, numbing, loss of feelings, or tendency to avoid reminders of a past traumatic event?
   a. Feeling a sense of detachment or restriction of range of emotions
   b. Avoiding thoughts, feelings, conversations, people, or activities that are reminders of past trauma
   c. Having memory lacunae/gaps with respect to past trauma-laden events
   d. Having a morbid view of the future (e.g., expected shortened length or outlook of remainder of health care career, life span, family life, etc.)
3. Do you have a heightened or exaggerated sense of arousal?
   a. Hyperalert or usually feeling "on guard"
   b. Pronounced startle reaction
   c. Irritability or a "short emotional fuse"
   d. Problems concentrating, sleeping, eating, or enjoying normal activities that previously brought you pleasure or provided a sense of mastery

4. Do you experience dramatic alterations in your outlook or world view?
   a. Personal sense of safety/trust is fragile
   b. Positive view of the human condition is absent
   c. View of one's own power, independence, and self-confidence/esteem is now questioned
   d. Awareness of cruelty or fragility of life (given the experiences of colleagues or patients whom you have treated) is often present in a depressing, somewhat frightening way
   e. Feelings of shame, guilt, depression, or worthlessness are increasingly present
5. Have you begun to demonstrate symptoms or exaggerated signs of antisocial/asocial behavior that were not present before the overwhelming/ongoing exposure to your patients' trauma?
   a. Dangerous behavior (e.g., sexual promiscuity, erratic/aggressive/careless driving patterns, fiscal irresponsibility, poor treatment plan development, etc.)
   b. Extreme irresponsibility in one's personal and professional lives
   c. Alcohol abuse, illegal drug use, self-medication, criminal behavior
6. Are your basic interpersonal relations becoming dramatically affected?
   a. Suspicious, cynical, or hypercritical style now present
   b. Boundary violations with patients and staff
   c. Loss of interest in activities at home and/or work
   d. Poor patterns of self-care resulting in alterations in interactions with others
   e. Lack of availability

The conditions included in this classification require exposure to a traumatic or stressful event including vicarious exposure as experienced by health professionals [i.e., therapists, medical and nursing professionals].)

The essential frame of reference to use in understanding this self-questioning is that having these symptoms is no more a sign of personal weakness than is having the symptoms of any medical disorder. This is important to note at the outset so that self-blame, self-debasement, or bravado does not prevent a careful self-examination—especially after a particularly difficult patient/clinical encounter. Working with young victims of abuse, pediatric oncology patients, victims of brutal rape, or severe burn patients over time would take a toll on anyone.

To ensure that the medical or nursing professional takes this approach, we point to these following general principles to keep in mind when seeking self-understanding after a single or series of traumatic encounters with patients.

1. Be as nonjudgmental and accepting of yourself as you would in dealing with those you care for who have undergone a traumatic event.
2. Constantly keep in mind that the symptoms you are experiencing as a result of the traumatic encounter are related to the experiences themselves rather than to an inherent personality weakness or lack of personality strength in oneself.
3. Know that when you are dealing with trauma on an ongoing basis as part of the work you do, then dealing with the symptoms and dangers of vicarious PTSD on an ongoing basis—rather than a once-and-for-all event—is to be expected.
4. Sharing your feelings and concerns with others is clinically wise; those who seek to go it alone either wind up leaving the field or acting out in unhealthy ways (alcoholism, overdetachment, promiscuity, etc.).
5. Grieving losses along with the family of patients (especially young persons) is a task that is periodically necessary for professionals in health care.

Another important factor in having a healthy attitude in dealing with *vicarious* PTSD in yourself is appreciating a bit more about PTSD in the general population, and it is to this topic that we turn next.

What Is Posttraumatic Stress Disorder?

Although we hear a lot about PTSD today—especially on the heels of the terrorism attack on the World Trade Center and the Pentagon and the overwhelming disruptions of the COVID-19 pandemic—it is far from a new phenomenon. A classic overview of the PTSD phenomenon is provided by Foy, Drescher, Fitz, and Kennedy:

> Surviving a life-threatening personal experience often produces intense psychological reactions in the forms of intrusive thoughts about the experience and fear-related avoidance of reminders. In the first few weeks following a traumatic experience these patterns are found in most individuals and thus seem to represent a natural response mechanism for psychological adaptation to a life-changing event. Persistence of this reaction pattern at troublesome levels beyond a three-month period, however, indicates that the natural psychological adjustment process, like mourning in the bereaved, has been derailed. At that point, the psychological reactions natural in the first few weeks become symptoms of PTSD. In other words, PTSD may be viewed as the persistence of a natural process beyond its natural time frame for resolutions.
>
> The cardinal features of PTSD are the trauma-specific symptoms of intrusion, avoidance, and physical arousal. The primary requirement is the presence of. . . . A life-threatening event, such as serious injury in a traffic accident, would satisfy this criterion, while the expected death of a loved one from natural causes would not. The current diagnostic system then groups PTSD symptoms into three additional categories. [It] includes the presence in some form of persistent intrusive thoughts and feelings. Recurrent distressing dreams or flashbacks while awake about the traumatic experience are examples. . . . [The second category] represents the presence of avoidance symptoms associated with the trauma, such as avoiding driving following a severe traffic accident or fear of sexual relations following sexual assault. More subtle forms of avoidance would be general numbing of responsiveness or the

absence of strong feelings about the trauma. . . . [The final] reflects the presence of symptoms of increased physical arousal and hyper-vigilance. Feelings of panic may be experienced in situations similar to the trauma; for example, combat veterans with PTSD may show powerful startle reactions to loud noises that resemble gunshots or explosions.

The medical history of PTSD can be traced back to studies of human reactions to trauma in the nineteenth century by German psychiatrists who discovered the similarities in the clinical courses of survivors of mining accidents and accidents which involved toxic exposure.[27] Two major developments at that time stimulated investigations into what was then called post-traumatic neurosis. The initial spark of medical interest in the subject was ignited by a series of wars, including the Civil War in America and the two World Wars in Europe. Early conceptions of combat-related PTSD by physicians working with veterans of World War I presented it as "shell shock," a consequence of organic dysfunction rather than a psychological process. This formulation arose from use in World War I of both chemical agents and explosives of a power that previously had been unimaginable.

The second impetus was the emergence of social programs in several countries which began to provide compensation for work-related or military service-related disabilities. The early description of traumatic reactions as "compensation reactions" referred to a perceived rise in numbers of victims seeking restitution after the first compensation laws were introduced in Europe. . . . This phenomenon presented an example of the tendency to relate symptoms of a trauma reaction to some process other than exposure to intense trauma itself.

While early views of post-traumatic reactions reflected the assumption that various types of trauma produced similar reactions, studies in the past twenty years have tended to be trauma-specific in their focus. Thus, labels for PTSD such as battle fatigue, rape trauma syndrome, and disaster survivor syndrome have developed in the literature [see Foa, Steketee, and Olasov Rothbam[28]] . However, most recently, studies have shown similarities among several survivor groups, including combat [see Foy, Sipprelle, Rueger, and Carroll[29] and Keane,

Fairbank, Caddell, and Zimering[30]] rape, domestic violence [see Houskamp and Foy[31]], childhood sexual abuse [see Briere[32]], childhood physical abuse [see Ammerman, Cassisi, Hersen, and Van-Hasselt[33]], transportation accidents [see McCaffrey and Fairbank[34]], and natural disasters [see Green, Grace and Gleser[35]; since 9/11, terrorism has been added to the list].

Common elements of traumatic experience include being physically and psychologically overwhelmed by a life-threatening event which is beyond the victim's prediction and control. To understand such complex reaction patterns requires the integration of findings from both biology and psychology. Thus, current perspectives on the nature of PTSD include contributions from several approaches, including biological, behavioral, cognitive [see Foa et al.[28]] and integrative [see Foy, Osato, Houskamp, and Neumann[36]].

From a biological perspective several studies in the past ten years have been conducted with Vietnam combat veterans with PTSD to examine their physiological reactions to combat trauma reminders or cues. Results from these studies have been consistent in showing large heart rate increases in most combat veterans with PTSD when they were exposed to combat cues. Other biological studies have also shown that combat veterans with PTSD have experienced changes in their central nervous systems so that they are overly sensitive to startle-producing noises. Studies are currently being conducted to determine whether these biological features are also applicable to PTSD associated with other types of trauma. Since these physical features of PTSD are almost universally described as painfully distressing in nature, this biological reactivity may be a critical element in the onset of social irritability and withdrawal in PTSD victims.

Contributions from behavioral psychology help in understanding how PTSD symptoms develop. Pavlovian conditioning occurs at the time of the trauma so that the overpowering feelings of life-threat and helplessness are paired with other cues present (which are not life-threatening). By this learning process these cues acquire the potential for evoking extreme fear when they are encountered later. The survivor also learns that escaping from these cues terminates the distressing fear.

Planning life activities to avoid painful reminders, an example of instrumental learning, may become a preferred coping strategy since it reduces the painful exposure to trauma reminders.

From a cognitive psychology perspective, the meaning which the survivor attaches to the traumatic experience may play an important role in PTSD. Perceptions of helplessness associated with the traumatic experience may serve to immobilize survivors' more active coping efforts, thereby serving to maintain PTSD symptoms.

While these approaches are helpful in explaining possible mechanisms for the development of PTSD, they do not explain why some individuals exposed to intense trauma do not develop enduring PTSD symptoms. To address this issue an integrative approach is necessary which includes additional factors beyond biological reactivity, Pavlovian and instrumental learning, and symbolic meaning. In our integrative model of PTSD, the experience of an overwhelming biological reaction during a life-threatening traumatic event lays the necessary foundation for the development of PTSD through behavioral and cognitive mechanisms of learning. However, other factors serve to mediate between exposure to trauma and the development of PTSD symptoms. Thus, an integrative approach to understanding PTSD includes the interaction between traumatic experiences and other non-trauma factors to account for the development or nondevelopment of PTSD [see Foy and Drescher, and Fitz[37]].

Knowing as much as you can about PTSD is essential not only for patient care and referral but also for your own health and the welfare of your colleagues and those who report to you. When vicarious PTSD disrupts medical and nursing professionals' frame of reference, the results will change one's world view; sense of professional and personal identity; and spiritual, psychological, and philosophical outlooks. The negative ripple effect may lead to personal alienation from friends and long-term coworkers and even in the relationship one has with oneself. It can cause an abrupt and inappropriate job change, a failed significant relationship and a dramatic alteration of one's personality style and approach to others (i.e., inability to modulate emotions). Extremes such as absenteeism or overinvolvement may not only cause personal problems but also may act as negative role modeling for other members of the treatment team.

The COVID-19 pandemic has exposed medical and nursing professionals to conditions that can lead to vicarious PTSD and other forms of secondary stress.

> The lessons of this pandemic have been painful; a health care system ill prepared to manage volumes of patients, short supplies of protective equipment to keep direct caregivers safe, job loss and economic stress not experienced since the Great Depression, isolation from loved ones, a constant barrage of information and speculation sometimes referred to as an "infodemic," and a lingering uncertainty about how long the pandemic will last and whether it will resurge. We are also witness to the enormous generosity of people who are finding creative ways to stay connected and live life as normally as possible, to the herculean efforts by scientists to understand the pathogenesis of COVID-19 and develop a vaccine and to the dedication of direct caregivers like nurses, physicians and first responders who risk their own health to care for those afflicted.[38p193]

The risks and problems endured during the COVID-19 pandemic have re-sensitized health professionals to the challenges of chronic secondary stress. And, building on this heightened awareness of the challenges of stress, knowing how to develop a self-care protocol, being able to increase one's ongoing level of self-understanding and self-awareness especially in difficult situations that may involve failure and loss of life, and knowing ways to strengthen one's inner life are also essential. Accordingly, it is to the topic of wicked problems, often the source of extreme stress, that we now turn.

References

1. Selye H. *The Stress of Life*. New York, NY: McGraw Hill; 1956.
2. Bode R. *First You Have to Row a Little Boat: Reflections on Life and Living*. New York, NY: Warner Books; 1995.
3. Dyrbye LN, Thomas MR, Huntington JL. Personal life events and medical student burnout: a multicenter study. *Academic Medicine*. 2006;81:374–384.

4. Eiser A. *The Ethos of Medicine in Postmodern America*. Lanham, MD: Lexington Books; 2014.

5. Clever L. Who is sicker: patients—or residents? Residents' Distress and the care of patients. *Annals of Internal Medicine*. 2002;136(5):391–393.

6. Auden WH. Introduction. In Hammarskjold D, ed. *Markings*. New York: Knopf; 1976:ix.

7. Coplan B, McCall TC, Smith NMA, Gilbert VL, Essary A. Burnout, job satisfaction, and stress levels of PAs. *Journal of the American Academy of Physician Assistants*. 2018;31(9):42–48.

8. Carpenter H. ANA's health risk appraisal: three years later. *American Nurse Today*. https://www.myamericannurse.com/wp-content/uploads/2016/12/ant1-NPWE-1219.pdf. Published January 2017. Accessed 6/18/2020.

9. Sanders L. *The Case of Lucy Bending*. New York, NY: Putnam; 1982.

10. Summers S, Summers HJ. *Saving Lives: Why the Media's Portrayal of Nursing Puts Us All at Risk*. New York: Oxford University Press; 2015.

11. Edelwich J, Brodsky A. *Burnout*. New York: Human Sciences Press; 1980.

12. Freudenberger H. Impaired clinicians: coping with burnout. In: Keller PS, Ritt L, eds. *Innovations in Clinical Practice: A Sourcebook*. Vol. 3 Sarasota, FL: Professional Resource Exchange; 1984.

13. United Nations. COVID-19 and the need for action on mental health. UN policy brief. https://unsdg.un.org/sites/default/files/2020-05/UN-Policy-Brief-COVID-19-and-mental-health.pdf. Published May 13, 2020. Accessed 6/25/2020.

14. Pfifferling JH. Cultural antecedents promoting professional impairment. In: Scott CD, Hawk J, eds. *Heal Thyself: The Health of Healthcare Professionals*. New York, NY: Brunner Mazel; 1986:3–18.

15. Gill J. Burnout: a growing threat to ministry. *Human Development*. 1980;1(2).

16. Wicks R. Countertransference and burnout in pastoral counseling. In: Wicks R, Parsons R, Capps D, eds. *Clinical Handbook of Pastoral Counseling*. Vol. 3 Mahwah, NJ: Paulist Press; 2003.

17. Gunderson L. Physician burnout. *Annals of Internal Medicine*. 135(201):145–148.

18. Halbesleben JRB, Rothert C. Linking physician burnout and patient outcomes: exploring the dyadic relationships between physicians and patients. *Health Care Management Review*. 2008;33(1):29–39.

19. Sotile WM, Sotile MO. *The resilient physician*. Chicago, IL: American Medical Association; 2002.

20. Sullivan P, Burke L. Results from CMA's huge 1998 physician survey point to a dispirited profession. *Canadian Medical Association Journal*. 1998;159:525–529.

21. Bean M. 84% of nurses have not been tested for COVID-19 and 5 other survey findings. *Becker's Hospital Review*. https://beckershospitalreview. Published May 4, 2020. Accessed May 22, 2020.

22. West CP, Dyrbye LN, Shanafelt TD. Physician burnout: contributing consequences and solutions. *Journal of Internal Medicine*. 2018;283;516–520.

23. American Nurses Association. Executive summary: ANA health risk appraisal findings. www.healthynursehealthynation.org. Published November 30, 2016.

24. Accreditation Review Commission on Education for the Physician Assistant. *Accreditation Standards for Physician Assistant Education*. Johns Creek, GA: ARC-PA; 2020.

25. Kottler J. *On Being a Therapist*. San Francisco, CA: Jossey-Bass; 1986.

26. Wicks R. *Riding the Dragon*. Notre Dame, IN: Sorin Books; 2002.

27. Kolb LC. A critical survey of hypotheses regarding posttraumatic stress disorders in light of recent research findings. *Journal of Traumatic Stress*. 1988;1(3):291–304.

28. Foa EB, Steketee G, Olasov Rothbam B. Behavioral/cognitive conceptualizations of post-traumatic stress disorder. *Behavior Therapy*. 1989;20:155–176.

29. Foy DW, Sipprelle RC, Rueger DB, Carroll EM. Etiology of posttraumatic stress disorder in Vietnam veterans: analysis of premilitary, military and combat exposure influences. *Journal of Consulting and Clinical Psychology*. 1984;52(1):79–87.

30. Foy DW, Sipprelle RC, Rueger DB, et al. Therapy reduces symptoms of PTSD in Vietnam combat veterans. *Behavior Therapy*. 1989;20:245–260.

31. Houskamp B, Foy DW. The assessment of PTSD in battered women. *Journal of Interpersonal Violence*. 1991;6(3):367–375.

32. Briere J. *Therapy for Adults Molested as Children: Beyond Survival*. New York, NY: Springer; 1989.

33. Ammerman RT, Cassisi JE, Hersen M, Van-Hasselt VB. Consequences of physical abuse and neglect in children. *Clinical Psychology Review*. 1986;6:291–310.

34. McCaffrey R, Fairbank J. Behavioral assessment and treatment of accident-related posttraumatic stress disorder: two case studies. *Behavior Therapy*. 1985;16:406–416.

35. Green BL, Grace MC, Gleser GC. Identifying survivors at risk: long-term impairment following the Beverly Hills supper club fire. *Journal of Clinical and Consulting Psychology* 1985;53:672–678.

36. Foy DW, Osato S, Houskamp B, Neumann D. Etiology factors in post-traumatic stress disorder. In: Saigh P, ed. *Posttraumatic Stress Disorder: A Behavioral Approach to Assessment and Treatment*. Oxford, England: Pergamon Press; 1992.

37. Foy D, Drescher K, Fitz A, Kennedy K. Post traumatic stress disorders. In: Wicks R, Parsons R, Capps D, eds. *Clinical Handbook of Pastoral Counseling.* Vol. 3. Mahwah, NJ: Paulist Press; 2003: 274–277.

38. Donnelly, G. From the editor: pandemic: looking back and thinking ahead. *Holistic Nursing Practice.* 2020;34(4):193–194.

Wicked Problems in Health Care

Identifying, Reframing, Sufficing, and Forgiving Oneself

Objectives

- Identify drivers of health care change that contribute to secondary stress.
- Differentiate between wicked and tame problems.
- Identify specific wicked problems in health care that lead to secondary stress.
- Differentiate between problem–solving and problem improvement.
- Describe dynamics of challenge, change and creativity in tackling wicked problems.

Some problems are so complex that you have to be highly intelligent and well informed just to be undecided about them.

—L. J. Peter

The CEO of a 600-bed regional hospital has invited the leadership of all clinical disciplines to a meeting. Nurses, physicians, physician assistants, and lab personnel begin to assemble. The mood in the room is upbeat, given that admissions for COVID-19 have been declining for 2 weeks and the situation is normalizing. The staff believes that the CEO has called this meeting to thank everyone for their herculean efforts and to give an update on the state of the hospital post COVID. Instead, the news was dire as he hesitantly explains.

"The Board of Directors has asked the hospital administration to begin a process of 'rightsizing' the clinical staff and to determine the

*best staffing and services mix to efficiently deliver the highest quality
care in light of the devastating revenue loses for elective procedures
during the last year. The board projects a 20% cut in staff in all major
clinical areas. I have called you together to solicit ideas on how to get
through this post-COVID period. Please put your recommendations
in writing and send to my office by Friday afternoon. We will recon-
vene to discuss the most promising recommendations and develop our
plan within the next 2 weeks." The CEO leaves before anyone asks
a question.*

*The room is silent at first. As staff file out, you listen to the chat-
ter in the hallway. Who will staff the units? What will staff patient
ratios be, especially in critical care? Suppose staff resign, and there is
a second wave of COVID-19? By the time the meeting disbands,
negative emotions were running high—so many questions, conflicting
perspectives, and outright fear. And then a voice from the center of the
staff expresses the group's anger and frustration, "Last week we were
heroes!" This hospital is experiencing a wicked problem catalyzed by
the COVID-19 pandemic dynamics and its unintended consequences.*

The term *wicked problem* originated in the design and planning literature. It slowly crept into the health care literature since it captures what
health professionals frequently experience in trying to solve problems
such as access to health care, reducing errors, coordination of care,
deconstructing and reconstructing medical and nursing education in a
technological age, and, most recently, dealing with a pandemic. Rittel,
an urban planner and designer, coined the terms *wicked* and *tame* problems to differentiate the solvability of problems encountered in his
field.[1] Tame problems

- have relatively clear definitions.
- generate stable problem statements.
- have stopping points or solutions that are either right or wrong.
- have solutions that can be tried or abandoned while the problem
  remains the same.
- belong to a class of similar problems that are usually solved in the
  same manner and can be directed by protocols.

Medical and nursing professionals are taught to diagnose and solve
problems using complex and systematic reasoning. When a patient presents with a specific problem/complaint, there are prescribed ways of

assessing the patient and using diagnostic tests. This process results in a diagnosis of the problem and a standard treatment that may be tailored to the individual patient. Even though many clinical problems create pain and suffering for the patient and can be difficult to diagnosis, they can be characterized as tame since they most often resolve when the correct intervention is applied. Solving problems for patients and families is a source of great personal satisfaction for health professionals. The process applied in such cases becomes second nature: assess, plan, intervene and evaluate. On the other hand, intervening in wicked problems is messy, produces no definitive answers, and is fraught with conditions that spawn new problems, promoting secondary stress for medical and nursing clinicians. There are no protocols or clinical rubrics for addressing such wicked problems. Accordingly, the wicked problem-solver will need perseverance, resilience, equanimity, and creativity to be successful. Further, the strategies discussed in other chapters that promote calm, introspection, clear thinking, spirituality, humor, and the ability to relinquish perfectionism are all necessary in any effort to grapple with wicked problems.

Analyzing Aspects of the COVID-19 Pandemic Through the Wicked Problem Lens

The characteristics of wicked problems, listed in the following text, are applied to the COVID-19 pandemic to illustrate the tangled and evolving complexity that promotes both primary and secondary stress in clinicians on the front lines of care.

> *Wicked problems are unique, often vague and defy definitive formulation especially since different individuals or groups see the problem situation from varying lenses, theories or even political perspectives which is referred to as "social complexity."*

The COVID-19 virus and the pandemic are unique in their expression. This SARS-related coronavirus (SARS-CoV-2) has defied previous notions of virus behavior and baffled the global scientific community. Drosten, a world-renowned virologist who has studied corona viruses for 17 years, expressed his surprise that coronavirus (COVID-19) emerged to be more deadly and much more transmissible than previous corona-type viruses. For example, it can spread from a host who is not experiencing symptoms.[2] COVID-19 is also now linked to a new syndrome that effects children's cardiac and respiratory systems, raising further questions concerning viral dynamics across the life span and with genetic and other individual variabilities.

Making matters worse, experts and political figures continue to offer conflicting theories and viewpoints about the origins of and approaches to the pandemic. And so, questions like the following abound:

• Did the virus emerge in a laboratory or in a "wet market" where animal meat is sold?
• Should everyone be tested or only those having symptoms?
• Are the diagnostic tests for COVID-19 reliable?
• Should all health care personnel be tested regardless of the presence of symptoms?
• Is the 14-day quarantine period sufficient for those who test positive?
• Who decides on the initiation of and process for contract tracing?
• Should tactics that promote "herd immunity" be used (i.e., mitigating social distancing measures and letting the virus run its course)?
• Should the wearing of masks be universally mandated or left to individual responsibility?

Medical and nursing personnel may also disagree on how to treat or provide care. For example, there have been conflicting views not only on testing but also on the effectiveness of drugs that might ameliorate symptoms. Early clinical trials validated the positive effects of Remdesivir, originally developed to treat Ebola, but will there be side effects and negative sequelae? Will there be enough of the drug available, and who will receive it?

Nesse[3] illustrates the inherent conflict that resides in the differences with which health care providers and administrators view and intervene in specific health care problems. He cites as an example, health care costs; "Providers think of patient compliance, preventive services and cost shifting. Payers think of excess utilization, provider strongholds, and waste. The government apparently thinks we haven't got enough regulations, and the patients think we (clinicians) are all at fault for the entire mess!"[3]

Among the general population, those who are believers in science and public health principles may conflict with those who believe in individual rights and the freedom to defy legislated measures designed to protect the public's health. There are also disagreements among medical and nursing professionals concerning the extent of their obligations to deliver care in environments that do not have sufficient protective equipment or staff. The question arises: Should they organize or just press on, caring for patients while risking health?

Clashing interprofessional viewpoints that conceptualize problems differently can be an enormous source of stress. The point here is that: *unique* problems with *unclear definitions generate* conflicting viewpoints and resultant *social complexity.* This social complexity can then deteriorate into dynamics of blame and finger-pointing exacerbating secondary stress for those involved. In summary,

> *wicked problems do not have final solutions. They are not problems that are definitively solved, like prescribing a proven drug for a common health problem. In fact, there are no solutions since wicked problems continue to morph into new, unique problems when attempts at solving are applied. Intervening in a wicked problem also produces unintended consequences that could be worse than what appeared to be the original problem.*

There is no better illustration of a wicked problem's *no-stopping rule* than a pandemic. History teaches that achieving "final control" of the virus or having "an end" to the cycles of infection will not happen, even if an effective vaccine is developed. A vaccine, hopefully, will confer some level of immunity in most individuals, but there is no guarantee. The virus may mutate multiple times and flourish in environments yet unknown. Consider the decades old common "flu," for which there is a vaccine but also an annual flu season with which we all live. During the 2018–2019 influenza season, the Centers for Disease Control and Prevention estimated that 35.5 million people got sick, 16.5 million visited a health provider for their illness. There were also 490,600 hospitalizations and 34,200 deaths of those who contracted influenza.[4]

Medical and nursing professionals are educated to "solve" clinical problems, yet wicked problems dictate that the word *solution* be removed from one's vocabulary. The notion of a clinical problem without a solution is difficult for clinicians. As Nesse, a physician, comments, "in our clinical practice all our patient problems have a stopping rule. They recover and go home. They transfer to another system, or they die. Health care system challenges are not going anywhere. We have discussed the many problems of *health care for all*, of my 31 years in practice, and we will be doing it for the next 310 years."[3] Nesse's approach is to select one aspect of a wicked problem and work to ameliorate it with the result of improving patient care and calmly facing the periodic storms.

After coming to grips with the "no stopping rule" there are the *"unintended consequences"* of specific interventions or attempts to "solve the problem." Consider the unintended consequences of "social distancing" such as loneliness, the anxiety of not seeing family or friends or not being able to visit the sick and dying. Those in clinical practice have reported living in hotels instead of at home to protect their families from possible infection. The rates of depression and suicide among medical and nursing professionals has increased through the pandemic as well.

Kupferschmidt points out that moving forward, "governments around the world must triangulate the health of their citizens, the freedoms of their population, and economic restraints. Can schools be reopened? Restaurants? Bars? Can people go back to their offices?"[5p218] These questions point to the inherent stress involved in possibly making the wrong call—in producing, unpredicted, *unintended consequences.*

For example, the pandemic has brought mass vaccinations for other diseases such as measles, polio, yellow fever, and cholera to a halt in poor countries. Berkley, the head of the global vaccine alliance, calls the dilemma, "A devil's choice"—to continue mass, door to door vaccination campaigns or move ahead and risk the spread of COVID-19.[6] Further, 23 countries have already suspended measles vaccinations that would have provided immunity for 78 million children. The *unintended consequences* of this decision are likely to be catastrophic. While the pandemic provides dramatic examples of wicked problem principles, think of the challenges with which clinicians regularly grapple in clinical settings. How many of them are wicked? How many attempts at resolution have resulted in a worsening of the situation, as well as in being blamed or criticized for the "failure to solve"? Table 2.1 illustrates how the mitigation strategy of social distancing produced a cascade of both positive and negative *unintended consequences.*

> *Wicked problems do not respond to the testing of a "definitive solution." The problem grows only better or worse as a function of attempts to intervene. There can be no absolute right or wrong or true or false answers as in tame problem-solving but there can be better or worse results as a function of intervention. Therefore, the problem*

Table 2.1 Unintended Consequences of Social Distancing/Lockdowns: A Pandemic Mitigation Strategy

Positive Unintended Consequences	Negative Unintended Consequences
1. Development of new technologies for screening and contact tracing	1. Major economic downturn because of business lockdowns.
2. Parents spending time with children.	2. Cancellation of elective procedures and delay of needed treatments.
3. Online learning proliferation and the develop of new learning technologies.	3. Decline of reimbursement to practices and hospitals.
4. Less driving, flying, and cleaner air.	4. Reckless driving as a function of light traffic.
5. Increased proficiency in the use of web-based meeting technologies.	5. Isolation, anxiety, loneliness, and depression.
6. Increase in the use of telehealth visits for primary care and counseling.	6. News/information overload.
7. Increased volunteerism and charitable giving.	7. Cancellation of summative celebratory events.

solver must embrace the mindset of "improvement" or "sufficing" in dealing with wickedness rather than one of complete cure or resolution.

It is difficult for clinicians to embrace a "sufficing" mentality. Medical and nursing practitioners prefer closure since they are educated to use complex processes and protocols to diagnose, intervene and evaluate *results*. Avoiding errors and adverse events as well as improving the quality of care are rationale for the systematization of diagnostic and intervention processes as well as for the design of "decision support systems" for clinicians. Yet, they do not always provide support.

Medical and nursing practitioners who hold management positions are often faced with additional wicked problems. Excessive time spent away from patient care, difficult staff or colleagues, inadequate and/or lagging reimbursement that creates financial stress, staffing patterns that do not match acuity, unrealistic expectations from senior management to make do with inadequate resources are challenges that managers must confront. Peterson reminds us:

Affordable quality health care in the United States is a wicked problem. So are economic disparity, racism, women's rights, homelessness and so on. As is any fractal piece of any of these. Mahatma Gandhi didn't completely "solve" his challenges of both independence and convincing Indians to live in harmony. Martin Luther King didn't solve his challenges. Neither have Gloria Steinem, Caesar Chavez, James Grant, or Malala Yousafzai. They all took on extremely wicked problems. And we live today in a better world because of their work. Hope and progress lie in the struggle forward.[7]

Understanding the concept of "wickedness," particularly the notion that some problems, like a virus, mutate and evolve, and are not subject to final resolution, can help the clinician come to terms with perfectionistic tendencies, overwhelming guilt and fear of failure that lead to anxiety, stress, and eventually burnout and traumatic stress.

At the end of a four-hour workshop, Wicked Problems in Nursing, the presenter was approached by one of the attending nurse managers who appeared to be on the verge of tears and who said:

> I had decided not to attend this workshop because I feared having to sit through another session that would make me feel even more inadequate. But the CNO said that attendance was mandatory for which I am now so grateful. There are several nagging problems I have been grappling with without much success. I have been beating myself up over what I believe to be my management failures. Today, as I applied the features of wicked problems to some of my management problems, I realized that I have been doing okay, creating improvements, some minor but some significant, two steps forward, one step back and a few to the side. I also realized that these problems, particularly staffing patterns and changing acuity and infection control, will need constant work, evaluation, and experimentation. I can't believe how free I feel, I hope it lasts.

In a span of four hours this nurse manager realized that replacing the "solving mentality" with the "sufficing mentality" could not only improve problem intervention processes and results in dealing with wicked problems but also reduce anxiety and feelings of defeat and inadequacy.

Wicked problems are usually symptomatic of other wicked problems in the system or at a higher system level; that is, high COVID-19 mortality rates among minorities may be a function of wide-ranging health disparities, a societal wicked problem.

Wicked clinical problems that have defied "solution" and have contributed to the complexity of care delivery in disruptive situations like pandemics can be responded to using a sufficing rather than a solving outlook. A "sufficing" mentality encourages clinicians to frame their efforts realistically and remain resilient in difficult situations. The following issues that meet the criteria for wickedness constitutes a web of interacting problems that conspire to produce frustration, stress, anxiety, and uncertainty for medical and nursing professionals:

- Health disparities.
- Co-morbidities.
- Decline in hospital capacity including the number of hospitals nationally and the dearth of hospitals in communities of great need.
- Inadequate health insurance and reimbursement creating financial stress for individuals and clinicians.
- Inadequate emergency preparedness including lack of personal protective equipment.
- The computerization of health care that deprives clinicians of time with patients.
- Post-COVID-19, the loss of health care positions and the abandonment of health care careers.

Given these difficulties, the psychological and conceptual tools in this book are designed to assist clinicians to practice self-care, to reframe wicked problems as gifts or challenges instead of burdens, to relinquish self-blame and guilt and to embrace challenges in ways to lead to improvements while recognizing that they may never be definitively "solved." Included in these difficulties is the question of "clinician guilt."

Wicks's[8] guide on managing such guilt through the pandemic offers perspective for health professionals who have and will live through disruptive, even disastrous situations. His suggestions are as follows.

Guilt and the Corona Virus

Nurses, physicians, physician assistants and other caregivers are now facing overwhelming odds and experiencing not only their own fears but also guilt. They must face not only patients who they cannot serve adequately because of a lack of resources but then must return home with the worry that they are infecting family, friends, and neighbors they encounter.

The psychological danger for them in these experiences is also to psychologically develop traumatic countertransference.

This occurs when we are faced with insurmountable odds and actually try to meet people's unrealistic expectations with the result that we feel guilt and even anger over our inability to meet them. When I was in Beirut working with helpers and healers they brought there from Aleppo, Syria so I could address them through an Arabic interpreter on resilience, you could see they were overwhelmed. They were experiencing significant traumatic countertransference because as caring persons they tried to meet the impossible demands of those who came for help.

When they encountered me, they then exhibited traumatic transference in which they projected onto me their sense of helplessness and hopelessness. They communicated this to me in many ways including sadness and anger. In essence, they were saying: "What can you do? You can never understand our plight dealing with so many needs while ISIS is breathing down our necks and we, too, are afraid."

In response, rather than reacting, I reflected first within myself that their negative feelings weren't about me—I wasn't that important. And then, with this reflection producing clarity, I reflected with them and in essence tried to communicate: "I have debriefed the relief workers evacuated from Rwanda after their genocide. I also was in Cambodia to help those trying to rebuild that country after years of terror and torture. I've also served as a Marine Corps Officer. But none of that really matters. I will never understand your unique situation and all the stresses you are under. However, as a specialist in the prevention of secondary stress (the pressures experienced in reaching out to others), you deserve to get whatever you can from my presentations and this time together so take what makes sense and leave the rest. You know best."

I then looked at their faces as I presented the material to see what they nonverbally seemed to find important. Much to my surprise the two things that seem to strike them deeply were friendship and prayer (or in secular terms, a sense of "mindfulness"). And so, I did what I could with these areas and the other information I presented and then did something essential if you are to remain faithful as a helper in overwhelming situations: I let go.

As a nurse, physician, physician assistant, psychologist, social worker, counselor, minister, and other caregiver, you can only do what you can with those you serve. You can only protect yourself physically as much as possible before returning home to those you love. If you step back from your role because of guilt, over-responsibility, or the anger and pain of your patients, this is understandable. Don't pick on yourself; you have given so much you don't deserve such bad treatment—especially from yourself!

On the other hand, if you can remain in the fray through keeping in mind and addressing the psychological dangers to you, you will be pure gift to those who need you—not simply for the physical care you offer but, of equal importance, in being able to remain with others when all you can provide is a sense of presence at a time when it is dark for patients, family, and even yourself. One of the greatest gifts you can share with others during those times is a sense of your own peace and a healthy perspective, but you can't share what you don't have. And so, be clear but also very gentle in how you view and treat yourself. Guilt is understandable at times but, in the end, it is a waste of energy and becomes problematic not simply for you but for those you serve and live with because the self is limited and when the resiliency reservoir is emptied, no one wins.[8]

These insights shared by Wicks resonate with the wisdom of Carlos Casteneda, who said, "The trick is in what one emphasizes. We either make ourselves miserable, or we make ourselves strong. The amount of work is the same." [9p221]

Problems as Gifts: The Reframing Process

The COVID-19 pandemic has presented unprecedented challenges to medical and nursing practitioners in an atmosphere of disagreement on best public health and treatment practices. This is largely driven by the novelty of the virus and the resultant social complexity which has created confusion, discord, and even lack of progress in managing the pandemic. On the other hand, the pandemic has

- stimulated creativity and innovation in managing large numbers of patients.
- improved the rapid manufacture and distribution of personal protective equipment and ventilators.
- prompted the discovery of technologies to detect, contact trace and mitigate risks of contracting the illness.
- renewed the focus on creating health buildings with proper ventilation, air quality, and light given the fact that individuals in the developed world spend 90 percent of their lives indoors.[10] (A World Green Building council report asserts that cognitive ability doubles as a function of well-ventilated offices and that nightly sleep time increases by 46 minutes when employees have windows in their work environments.[10])

In China, where the pandemic has evolved, the use of temperature-detection technologies, wearables, and apps are now employed to immediately identify those who are risk of spreading the virus. Also, in some Chinese hospitals, robots are delivering meals, collecting used linens and trash and in some cases delivering medications. Drones are now available to deliver parcels and spray disinfectant as well.[11] Those who have the courage to innovate, to embrace challenges during a crisis such as a pandemic, and to employ cognitive flexibility and reframing are serving patients and front-line clinicians and creating healthier work environments.

Reframing and Problem-Solving

In the classic work on change and problem resolution, Watzlawick et al. defined reframing as a cognitive process by which the individual intentionally changes the meaning of a situation they have experienced.[12] There are three principles involved: first, we experience the world based on how we have learned to categorize experiences—for example, glass half empty (pessimist) or half full (optimist). Second, we recognize it is difficult to change these conceptual patterns since they are ingrained and automatic. Finally, we develop the ability to change our conceptual patterns or mindsets and see a situation in an alternate frame. The overarching goal of this approach is to free ourselves from our own conceptual traps.

As Watzlawick explains; "what turns out to be changed as a result of reframing is the meaning attributed to the situation, and therefore its consequences, but not its concrete facts."[14p95] For example, we can deliberately change the meaning we attribute to a situation, like, "The hospital administration is out to get us again," to "The hospital administration is struggling to see their way through this, let's see what we can do to help." When we approach the problem in this fashion, the goal is to alter our perspective to reduce our level of anger, reactivity, and distress. In the first century CE, the philosopher Epictetus observed, "It is not the things themselves that trouble but the opinions that we have about these things."[13] Shakespeare in the 17th century wrote in a similar vein that "there is nothing either good or bad, but thinking makes it so."[1] In the 20th century, Mark Twain gave his character, Huckleberry Finn, the gift of reframing as Finn convinced his friends that whitewashing the fence was fun instead of drudgery and all were eager to participate.[14] Finally, Hanh,[15] a modern Buddhist teacher, tells the story of the arrow—when the arrow strikes, the initial pain is intense. However, the second arrow, one's reaction to the pain including fear, anger, or despair can be even worse, magnifying the suffering. Medical and nursing practitioners may experience difficulties at work and spin negative theories about the motivations of colleagues and of those in charge thus exacerbating their own negative emotions often leading to chronic stress. Reframing can be a useful cognitive strategy in relinquishing self-blame and blaming others and in rekindling the joy in tackling problems and improving work and life.

Humor and imagination can also be freely employed in the reframing process since with wicked problems there is nothing to lose, there are no definitive solutions only possible improvements. While it may seem trite, having fun while engaging in the identification and exploration of wicked problems can free up cognitive processes and prevent stupidity, a state of mind that is more reflective of cognitive rigidity than lack of intellectual ability. Intelligence and stupidity often co-exist in certain individuals. As Welles[16] asserts, stupidity is the inability to adjust one's cognitive schemas to the everchanging contingencies of reality. The process outlined in Box 2.1 will assist in not only loosening cognitive

---

1. *Hamlet* (1603), Act 2, Scene 2, p. 11.

Box 2.1 A 12-Step Process for Identifying and Intervening in Wicked Problems

1. Write a 1-paragraph description of the problem with which you have been grappling. Include the length of time you have been dealing with the problem. Give the problem a short name (e.g. Low Staff Morale; Recurring Patient Infections).

2. Convene a meeting of work colleagues and share only the name you have assigned to the problem. Ask each colleague to write a short description of the problem you have named.

3. Ask each person to read their description of the problem, noting similarities and differences.

4. Review the characteristics of wickedness and evaluate the nature the problem under discussion. If the problem is deemed tame, set the goal and specify the interventions. If the problem is deemed wicked proceed with the following.

5. Describe past attempts at intervening in the problem and the results.

6. Describe how the problem has morphed; that is, write a new description of the problem postintervention noting any changes.

7. Describe the staff's responses to interventions (i.e., positive, negative, neutral) and the emotional pitch of the workgroup.

8. Discuss what the wicked problem may be symptomatic of in the work unit, in the organization, in health care in general?

9. Identify the positive and negative unintended consequences of interventions attempted.

10. Identify what the problem interventions have cost in both quantitative and qualitative terms.

11. Describe several scenarios, post intervention, with which the work group can live.

12. Identify spin-off problems and possible interventions that may lead to a more effective work environment and contribute to the larger organization.

If all problem definitions are relatively the same, the problem may be tame. Decide on a solution and test it. Move toward some agreement and proceed with a plan of action since "solution" is impossible and then evaluate results produced by the plan of action. Keep at it!

schemas but also in determining the degree of problem wickedness and the effectiveness of intervention strategies that lead to sufficing.

The education of clinical professionals emphasizes stepwise processes and standard protocols to diagnose and select interventions and to essentially solve tame problems. Understanding the concept of wickedness gets the clinician back to reality,

- Where a syndrome can look very different from patient to patient,
- Where an infection control process, however detailed and explicit, can fail because the infecting agent is not well understood, and
- Where a group of clinicians have very divergent views of "the problem" and how to manage it.

Conklin succinctly captures how failure to embrace the concept of wickedness can increase chaos, social complexity, and secondary stress in any work environment.

In times of stress the natural human tendency is to find fault with someone else. We tend to take the problem personally, at an organizational level, and assume that the chaos we see is a result of incompetence or, worse, insincere leadership. Since our education and experience have prepared us to see and solve tame problems, wicked problems sneak up on us and create chaos. Without understanding the cause, there is finger-pointing instead of learning.[17pp21–22]

The next chapter will address self-reflection and self-knowledge so that we can more effectively explore the roots of conflict in ourselves and in our clinical practice relationships and environments. Self-reflection and self-knowledge will enhance our problem solving abilities, particularly when dealing with wicked problems.

References

1. Rittel HWJ, Webber MM. Dilemmas in a general theory of planning. *Policy Sciences.* 1973;4:155–169.
2. Kupferschmidt K. The Coronavirus czar. Science. 2020;368(6490):462–465.
3. Nesse R. A wicked problem: Health care system reform and change. *Council of Accountable Physician Practices.* https://accountablecaredoctors.org/health-care-reform/a-wicked-problem-healthcare-system-reform-and-change/. Published 2014. Accessed May 9, 2020.
4. Center for Disease Control and Prevention. Estimated influenza illnesses, medical visits, hospitalizations, and deaths in the US 2018–19 influenza season. https://www.cdc.gov/flu/about/burden/2018-2019.html. Published January 8, 2020. Accessed May 11, 2020.
5. Kupferschmidt K. The lockdown worked, but what comes next. *Science.* 2020;368(6488):218–219.
6. Roberts L. Pandemic brings mass vaccinations to a halt. *Science.* 2020;368(6487):116–117.
7. Peterson T. Health in America is a wicked problem. *Stakeholder Health.* https://stakeholderhealth.org/wicked-problem/. Published January 20, 2016. Accessed May 12, 2020.
8 Wicks R. Guilt and facing the coronavirus: A guide for professional helpers and healers experiencing traumatic countertransference. Nursing 2020. Headlines. Friday, March 20, 2020, https://journals.lww.com/nursing/blog/intouch/pages/post.aspx?PostID=122. Accessed September 27, 2020.
9. Castaneda C. *Journey to Ixilan: The Lessons of Don Juan.* New York, NY: Simon and Schuster; 1972.
10. Helm D. The healthy building movement: A focus on occupants. *Floor Daily.* https://www.floordaily.net/floorfocus/the-healthy-building-movement-a-focus-on-occupants-augsep-2017. Published 2017. Accessed May 14, 2020.
11. Luo H, Galasso A. The one good thing caused by COVID-19: Innovation. *Working Knowledge: Harvard Business School* https://hbswk.hbs.edu/item/the-one-good-thing-caused-by-covid-19-innovation. Published May 7, 2020. Accessed May 12, 2020.
12. Watzlawick P, Weakland J, Fisch R. *Change: Principles of Problem Formation and Problem Resolution.* New York, NY: W. W. Norton; 1974.

13. Epictetus. *The Enchiridion.* http://classics.mit.edu/Epictetus/epicench. html Published 135 BCE. Accessed May 14, 2020.

14. Twain M. *The Adventures of Huckleberry Finn.* Project Guttenberg E-book #76. https://www.gutenberg.org/files/76/76-h/76-h.htm. Original work published 1885. Last updated May 25, 2018. Accessed May 14, 2020.

15. Hanh TN. *No Mud, No Lotus.* Berkeley, CA: Parallax Press; 2014.

16. Welles JF. *The Story of Stupidity.* Orient, NY: Mt. Pleasant Press; 1988.

17. J. Conklin. Wicked problems and social complexity. 2001–2005, *Cognexus Institute.* https://cognexus.org/wpf/wickedproblems.pdf. Revised October 8, 2008.

THREE

"Riding the Dragon"

Enhancing Self-Knowledge and Self-Talk in the Health Care Professional

Objectives

- Recognize the role of reflection in developing healthy perspective in the professional role.
- Explore how clinical professional stereotypes impede healthy and effective interactions.
- Identify the types of transferences that occur between patients and clinicians and among clinicians from diverse healthcare disciplines.
- Identify personal agendas, body signals, and irrational ways of thinking as a prelude to more effectively managing stress.
- Conduct a self-assessment using the questionnaire for medical and nursing professionals.
- Explore the roots of conflict in ourselves and in clinical practice roles.

The unexamined life is not worth living.

—Aristotle

Dr. Jones was finally completing his documentation at the end of a 12-hour shift. He imagined crashing on one of the cots set up in the doctor's lounge when the chief resident appeared and silently glared at him for what seemed to be a very long time. Finally, the words began to pour out —clipped and deliberate at first—then rapidly demanding.

"We will assume you went to school . . . and that they taught you to read English, at some point! That order is written in English," he said, angrily pointing to the page. "Now give the patient the medication before he dies!" he shouted as he backed into the elevator." Embarrassed and angry, Dr. Jones did not respond; he did not have time. He gave the medication, left the unit, and finally crashed in the break room—but he could not sleep.

Enhancing Self-Knowledge and Self-Talk in the Health Care Professional

In a foreword to a book on identifying and avoiding defensive patterns in working with patients, Dame Lesley Southgate wrote, "The missing pieces about the failure of some doctors to incorporate best practice into the consultation may be addressed by paying attention to what the doctor is feeling rather than what he/she knows."[1pviii] This advice also applies to identifying and avoiding defensive patterns in working with colleagues no matter your clinical discipline. If acute and chronic secondary stress is to be limited and one's personal and professional well-being is to be enhanced, self-knowledge and the enlightened behavior that it should give rise to are not a nicety in medical/nursing practice; they must be a given. Personal discipline and self-control are essential in medicine and nursing, as they are for all professionals responsible for the care for others. In the behavioral sciences, this is referred to as "self-regulation." In a book for psychologists on self-care, Baker writes, "*Self-regulation,* a term used in both behavioral and dynamic psychology, refers to the conscious and less conscious management of our physical and emotional impulses, drives and anxieties."[2p15] She then goes on to warn:

> Managing our affect, stimulation, and energy as we navigate our professional and personal lives, as well as our relationships with self and others, is no easy task. To regulate mood and affect, we must learn how to both proactively, constructively manage dysphoric affect (such as anxiety and depression) and adaptively defuse or "metabolize" intense, charged emotional experiences to lessen the risk of becoming emotionally flooded and overwhelmed.[2p15]

In the story that opens this chapter, the chief resident and resident were no doubt running on automatic pilot, instead of engaging in any form of conscious self-regulation. However, as Coster and Schwebel point out, if we are to "manage" ourselves or "regulate" our behavior, obviously sound self-awareness must be present.[3] Nowhere is this more necessary than in clinical settings.

Self-awareness is especially important for persons working in high-stress settings that require great intelligence and high standards. In such professions, "perfectionism and its associated demon, fear of failure," as Block recognizes, can be quite dangerous to persons attracted to health care.[4pviii] He goes on to point out the following:

> Health professionals are held, and for the most part hold themselves, to extremely high standards of performance. It is believed that they should always be at the peak of technical proficiency, emotionally available, straightforward, clear, and compassionate. The rewards for this are high status, admiration, and respect. Lapses are in two directions: cynicism and money grubbing, or despair, feelings of failure, and disgrace. This latter triad is often associated with the more frank and overt symptomatic breakdown into addiction and substance abuse.[4pix]

It is very easy to lose one's way—even from the very beginning of one's journey in professional health care. Unfortunately, this problem does not end with graduation and entry into practice. Loss of perspective remains a danger throughout one's career if time is not taken to reflect on one's personal and professional lives. The following anecdote on how easy it was for a seasoned neurologist to lose a sense of what was important illustrates this well. He demonstrates, that sometimes even when you are dealing with life and death on a daily basis, it takes someone from your circle of friends or family to shock you into reality and remind you how quickly all of us can blow things out of proportion when we do not take time out to reflect on our feelings, thoughts, beliefs, and behavior.

> The following letter, written by a first-year college student to her father during the middle of her second semester, delightfully points (out how easy it is to lose perspective no matter how delicate and important one's work is). Prior to receiving this note, her father was totally preoccupied with her "success" in college. He was worried because she didn't do well

in her first semester and was concerned, she would fail out during the second semester—and take his money with her! He had forgotten, as many of us parents do, that performance in courses is only a partial measure of learning; moreover, there is much more to the total college experience than just grades.

Despite her youth, this woman knew this better than he, and so taught him an important lesson on perspective. On the front page of her note it said:

Dear Dad,

Everything is going well here at college this semester, so you can stop worrying. I am very, very happy now . . . you would love Ichabod. He is a wonderful, wonderful man and our first three months of marriage have been blissful.

And more good news Dad. The drug rehab program we are both in just told us that the twins that are due soon will not be addicted at birth.

Having read this, her father then turned the page with trepidation. On the other side of the note it said:

Now, Dad, there actually is no Ichabod. I'm not married nor pregnant. And I haven't ever abused drugs. But I did get a "D" in chemistry, so keep things in perspective![5p115]

It is very easy to move through life—even the most service oriented of lives—in such a compulsive, driven way that we feel out of control. When we take out time to reflect on who we are, what we are doing, we often get a glimpse of the roots of our behavior, realizing how "unfree" we have become in so many ways. The bottom line is that you can count on losing perspective and deluding yourself if time is not devoted to reflection on your thoughts, behavior, and affects. But it is not easy to be honest with yourself.

Zen master Shunryu Suzuki once cautioned his students, "When you are fooled by something else, the damage will not be so big. But when you are fooled by yourself, it is fatal" (cited in Chadwick[6p308]). In health care, this is a particular danger. DeChant and Shannon[7] point out that the medical profession does little to emphasize self-care.

> Rather is creates the expectation that the norm is long workdays, insufficient time to re-energize, and little opportunities for personal activities. This aspect of the culture . . . combined with the personality trait of compulsiveness, may reduce

the likelihood that physicians will prioritize stress reduction techniques.[7pp44-45]

This observation can be extended to most medical and nursing professionals.

An interprofessional team of clinicians formed a study group to review research findings on the effectiveness of COVID-19 screening tests for both the virus and for antibodies. The studies' findings did not offer a clear directive on test accuracy particularly with respect to antibodies. There was much debate on the quality of the studies and the interpretation of the findings. The group decided to proceed with their current protocol and continue to monitor research findings.

This detailed review of research studies is something we applaud and possibly expect of medical and nursing professionals who are taught in their educational programs to review available evidence. However, it is only recently that medical and nursing professional associations and educational programs are attending to the alarming evidence and promoting self-assessment and self-care for health professionals as essential curricular content. Further, the pandemic is confronting health professionals with their lack of self-knowledge, deficiencies in self-care, and fragile resilience.

Attaining self-knowledge, the foundation of self-care, is sometimes elusive, even if one pursues psychotherapy. Donald Brazier reflects this reality in a book advocating the use of an integration of Zen with psychotherapy when he notes,

These days . . . we are apt to seek out a therapist to . . . help us get the dragon back into its cave. Therapists of many schools will oblige in this, and we will thus be returned to what Freud called 'ordinary unhappiness' and, temporarily, heave a sigh of relief, our repressions working smoothly once again. Zen, by contrast offers dragon-riding lessons, for the few who are sufficiently intrepid.[8p14]

Given the personal psychological dangers to medical and nursing practitioners and their patients when they are not self-aware, they must be among those who are "the sufficiently intrepid" with respect to self-awareness. To deal with simple self-mentoring and to learn to "ride the dragon," approaches using cognitive and psychodynamic psychology are provided here for consideration.

Uniqueness and Self-Knowledge

No matter what approach is used to understand stress—be it weighted in the direction of environment or personality—the individual is always a major factor. This is observable in persons who seek psychiatric or psychological treatment. We have found the following:

> A significant turning point in therapy or counseling arrives when the individual seeking help is able to grasp the follow-ing, simple, seemingly paradoxical reality: When we truly accept our limits, the opportunity for personal growth and development is almost limitless. Prior to achieving this insight, energy is wasted on running away from the self, or running to another image of self.[9pp5-6]

Such obviously is the case with most of us. This should not be sur-prising. Poets, theologians, and great scientists have joined those in the mental health field to warn people to not be unconsciously pulled into trying to be someone you are not. In the words of e.e. cummings, for example, "To be nobody but yourself in a world which is doing its best, night and day, to make you everybody else—means to fight the hard-est battle which any human being can fight, and never stop fighting."[10]

The point here is that it can be a great struggle to be "simply our-selves" to do what is really best for ourselves especially when we are in a transferential role such as physician, nurse, or physician assistant where patients, colleagues or managers are turning to us as the "designated helpers" in ways they turned to parents and significant figures from the past.

Consider the following case:

> *A seasoned staff nurse in an employee health clinic is preparing for the pre-summer rush of new employees. The new clinic director fre-quently makes statements such as, "I wish I had someone to . . ." or "If I only had time to . . ." or "This report is taking so much of my time . . ." which prompts the nurse to automatically volunteer to help. The staff nurse is frustrated with the director whom she believes*

is taking advantage of her. She vows to "tell him off" but never does. Instead each day the cycle begins anew despite self-promises to change behavior. After some guided self- assessment, the nurse realizes that she has willingly conformed to her own image of "chronic helper," a role often assumed by nurses. Instead of succumbing to her self-imposed helpfulness, she does not respond immediately to the director's prompts. If he makes a direct request like report writing, she offers her files for his use in preparing the report. Eventually the nurse is acting based on the reasonableness of direct requests rather than to "hints" that tap into her "inner helper."

These situations are common, but in terms of our own sense of self, we must be aware that this perception of "health care professional as perennial helper" is based on the needs and personality of the other, on our own faulty self-images and not on our abilities or objective reality. Being "extraordinary" is not being a super-person who attends to all requests, even hints, and meets all needs as some (including, unfortunately, some of our colleagues) want us to believe. Instead, it is being self-aware and in tune with the way our talents and the needs of those with whom we work in health care act in synchronicity. Accomplished inventor and global citizen R. Buckminster Fuller phrased it this way in terms of his own life and the dangerous lures he met during his life:

> The only important thing about me is that I am an average healthy human being. All the things I've been able to do, any human being, or anyone, or you, could do equally or better. I was able to accomplish what I did by refusing to be hooked on a game of life that had nothing to do with the way the universe was going. I was just a throwaway who was willing to commit myself to what needed to be done. (cited in Wicks[11p6])

Resonating with Fuller's view takes a degree of humility. Yet, with such humility, health care professionals can avoid the unnecessary stress that comes from living as if the transferences put on them by patients, colleagues, and managers are in fact a reality. Further, health professional students, who seasoned practitioners are called to guide, also benefit. In his discussion of humility among medical educators, Pfifferling, rightly indicates,

> Students can be exposed to the mistakes made by their faculty so that error in problem solving can improve learner behavior.

Faculty self-disclosing behavior and modeling of personal/ professional humility to a student reinforce the necessity to be on guard against medical arrogance that can cost a patient his life. By self-disclosing mistakes to their students, the faculty prevent the student from becoming too arrogant or too distanced from the troubles of their patients, and provider/patient bonding is strengthened and improved.[11p14]

Humility and its connection with emotional sensitivity on the part of medical and nursing professionals therefore is not a sign of weakness. Instead, humility is a sign of balance, self-awareness, and maturity that raises the quality of interactions between patient and caregiver and between caregiver and colleagues. Coombs and Fawzy's insights on medical education extends to the education of all health professionals in that such education usually emphasizes only the "hands" (technique) and the "head" (knowledge) and fails to explore the role of the "heart" (emotional sensitivity), which also includes an acceptance of one's failures.[12] Thus, it diminishes not only the quality of the clinician's own life but also the quality of patient care and the mentoring of new practitioners.[12p14]

Full self-awareness that includes an appreciation of our emotional sensitivity or lack of it is very elusive. In the words of poet Henry David Thoreau, "it is as hard to see oneself as to look backwards without turning round" (cited in Auden[13pix]). Yet, every effort must be made to increase self-understanding—not just to curb our errors but also to increase our self-respect because as Leech aptly notes, " "You do not want to know someone whom you despise, even if, especially if, that someone is you."[14pp43–44] Self-awareness and self-respect feed each other and form a positive circle. Self-respect *is* true self-awareness.

To become clearer about ourselves, there is a need to expend energy, but it obviously helps to know the most productive and efficient way to do this. To best accomplish a sense of clarity about our feelings, beliefs, and actions, appreciating the value of discipline, noting inconsistencies and exaggerated emotions, and avoiding vagueness (a sign that the defense of unconscious repression is at work) would be helpful and can be a lifelong process. A nurse's personal approach to this process is described in Box 3.1.

Box 3.1 A Nurse's Musings on Seeking Self Knowledge

Self-reflection, self-assessment, and self-critique can be difficult processes. Working with patients with mental disorders as
well as with health professionals in stress management work-
shops, necessitated my own periodic trips to the well of self-
understanding. To overcome the resistances we all experience in
working on the self, I engaged in a variety of psychotherapeu-
tic modalities to facilitate my own development. For example,
I have been through didactic group therapy twice which is a
process by which one gleans not only the rationale and meanings of one's group behavior but the overall dynamics of how
groups form and operate. I then moved to psychodrama where
a Moreno-trained psychodrama leader facilitated the group in
selecting a life drama from each of the participants, oversee-
ing the selection of protagonists and antagonists for the drama,
directing the drama and then conducting the de-briefing in
which each group member offered their own interpretations
and self-insights. In one session, I was chosen as the only meaningful figure in the life of a person who struggled mightily with
isolation and loneliness. I was selected to be her beloved dog
and spent the duration of the drama, lying at her feet. I learned
so much about the dynamics of loneliness and about staying
silently supportive.

My most intensive and long-term self-care experience was
10 years of psychotherapy with a phenomenological psycho-
analyst, every week for one hour and I never missed a session.
I entered this process at the urging of my adolescent daughter
who believed I would benefit, "because, Mom, you are nuttier
than I am." And so, I took the dare and the timing was impec-
cable since I struggled with leaving a leadership position that
I had held for 17 years. Unfortunately, my new employer landed
in bankruptcy a year after I arrived. It was the most stressful time
in my career not knowing if the University and the School that
I was leading would even survive—but we did and then I had
to contend with the stressors of merging into a new university

culture. I do not think I would have fared as well as without those weekly psychotherapy sessions. There is nothing quite like having the undivided attention of someone who listens deeply, questions supportively and challenges with care. I learned so much about myself; especially my proverbial buttons and what pushes them. I also search in books to give me perspective. Over the past decades I have gravitated to the Eastern literature particularly Zen Buddhist and Tao writings. There are certain books I keep close to my desk like *The Mind of Clover* by Robert Aitken and *No Mud, No Lotus* by Thich Nhat Hanh. One of my most important learnings from Zen is that you cannot prevent adversity in your life but you can shape your reactions to it and enrich your perspective and ways of responding to the next stressful life event—which is guaranteed to happen.

Embarking on a Disciplined Search

Self-awareness is an ongoing, dynamic undertaking that requires daily attention. With such a process in place, we can become more attuned to the rhythms of our personality and have our "psychological fingers" on the pulse of where we are emotionally with respect to an issue, a person, a challenge, or the general thrust of where our life is moving.

To accomplish this, we need to be aware of the ebb and flow of our reactions so we can become more sensitive to the subtle inconsistencies in our affect (i.e., experiences of sadness, depression, happiness, etc.), cognitions (ways of thinking, perceiving, and understanding), and bodily responses to potential stress and actions. This awareness provides us with a link to some of the motivations and mental agendas that lie just beyond our awareness—what some would refer to as our "preconscious." To be in a position for such an appreciation of ourselves, time must be taken to identify anything in the way we live that is incongruent so we can seek to understand the reason for the difference.

Instead, what often happens when we do, think, or feel something that is generally out of character for us is that we dismiss it as irrelevant or excuse it ("I was just tired, just having a bad day"). However, when we do not seek to accomplish a creative synthesis in understanding all parts of ourselves, we miss the normally buried treasures in our psyche that we might draw upon when living through difficult situations.

Elements of Clarity

One of the constants present when health care professionals seek help to avoid or limit the sources and symptoms of secondary stress is the temporary lack of clarity they are experiencing. In mentoring, the goal is to help them to clarify, to discern different approaches, and to problem-solve, to find solutions to their inner and external stresses. To accomplish this, time must be taken to focus on the specifics of their reactions. This helps the person to move through conscious (suppression) and unconscious/preconscious (repression) avoidance or forgetting. By limiting vagueness and a tendency to generalize or gloss over details and feelings, information that lies just beyond our sense of awareness becomes available. So, rather than turning away from the seemingly unacceptable feelings, cognitions, impulses, and reactions, we face the resultant anxieties as a price for learning more about ourselves. The benefit, of course, is greater self-knowledge and, in turn, more personal freedom. Rather than being limited by our blind spots in self-awareness and the waste of energy on defensiveness, by focusing on our daily interactions we seek to become sensitive to *all* of our reactions—even the seemingly incongruous ones—as a way to deepen self-knowledge.

Resistance to achieving clarity in life is often a function of limiting our focus on the roles and behavior of others (e.g., patients, their families, or our colleagues), and denying our own actions. We also must examine our *own* behavior, cognitions, and affect. *Clarity is a process by which we must be willing explore how we might be denying, minimizing, rationalizing, or hiding things from ourselves.* Although we may believe that we desire to see ourselves and our situation as they truly are, conflict can arise when this happens because the responsibility then falls on us to

- Become more aware of our own agendas—including the immature ones.
- Increase self-awareness of our body's responses to potential stress.

- Find appropriate levels of intimacy with those with whom we interact.
- Learn from our negative emotions, our defensiveness, and tendencies to project blame onto others.
- Recognize failure as opportunity and deal with anger and unhelpful reactions to failure.
- View ourselves and stressful situations from a lens of humor.
- Achieve a level of skill as a critical thinker.
- Overcome resistances to change.
- Improve self-talk as we reach for clarity.

Awareness of Our Agendas

Thinking that we do things for only one reason is naïve. In most cases, there are numerous reasons—some immature, some mature—that we do things. Because the reasons we do not like to acknowledge often remain beyond our awareness, clarity calls us to embrace all of them. In this way, the immature reasons can atrophy, and the mature ones can grow and deepen. However, to accomplish this goal, we must first accept that we are all defensive in some unique way. Such an admission is an excellent first beginning because it does not put us in the position of asking, "Are we, or aren't we?" Instead, it moves it out of the black-and-white situation to the gray areas where most of us live psychologically. When we look at all the reasons why we reacted to a situation in the way we did, we can begin to appreciate why people react to us in the way that they do. Otherwise, we remain puzzled, feel misunderstood, and project the blame outward so as never to learn what are the dynamics and how to unravel them in any given situation.

For instance, if colleagues do not like to work with us in stressful situations, it would be helpful for us to know what they are seeing so that we can work on adjusting or changing our behavior. A candidate applying for an administrative position asked her future supervisor, the department chair, during the interview, "Do you know how human resources is billing the main challenge of working with you?" Surprised—in considering how there could be *any* challenge in working with him? The department chair responded, "No,

I don't." To which she noted with a smile, "They are billing you as a perfectionist who gives vague instructions and gets upset when they are not followed exactly." The department chair continued with the interview.

Impatience, anger, and other reactions on our part do not increase efficiency when we are working with colleagues in a difficult health care emergency. Blaming our reactions solely on other people's incompetence provides very limited information for improving the situation by changing our own behavior. Even if the others were not as prepared as they should have been to handle, for example, a patient care situation, reacting emotionally or blaming others in a way that makes the situation deteriorate further, certainly does not improve things.

Clarity calls us to recognize our agendas, face our own fears, understand the games we play with others, lessen our defensiveness, develop new coping skills, and create alternative ways to deal with stressful situations. As Aitken points out, "it is only when we can generously acknowledge our own dark side and the shining side of the other, that you can be said to be truly on the path."[15p76] Yet, to do this, we need to be honest. We must appreciate that this honesty can have a positive domino effect in our life as a way of moving through the resistances we have to growth and change. When we start focusing on understanding individual interactions, larger questions open up as to whether we are getting enough rest or leisure, the right balance of time alone and with good friends, and how and when we are setting limits in all aspects of our life. It is important to recognize that the self is a limited entity that can be depleted if we do not involve ourselves seriously in a process of self-care.

Awareness of the Body's Responses

The Buddhist teacher Thich Nhat Hanh reminds us, "If we get in touch with our body, then we can also get in touch with our feelings."[16] The tendency, however, is to experience a negative event which prompts bodily signals that we often ignore. We then think, even ruminate about what happened creating a second painful perspective which Hanh refers to as the second arrow.

The unwelcome things that sometimes happen in life – being rejected, losing a valuable object, failing a test . . . are analogous to the first arrow. They cause some pain. The second arrow, fired by our own selves, is our reaction, our storyline, and our anxiety. All these magnify the suffering. Many times, the ultimate disaster we're ruminating upon hasn't even happened.[15p46]

Attuning to body signals can be helpful in assessing our true responses to situations and in developing responses that match the situation. Table 3.1 lists typical body responses to stressful situations that you may experience. You may be surprised, even concerned, about how long you had to think before deciding on the items to check. You may be aware of only global feelings but focusing on the specific signal will lead to a realization of just how the body's response influences your behavior.

Once we begin to link body signals to the feelings experienced in negative reactions, we are better able to accept the signal, interpret it, and perhaps reinterpret to our advantage and devote energy to responding more effectively. Your body is a mind-reader, but your mind can generate new meanings to experiences that can ultimately change your body's responses. This body–mind cycle can be enormously productive in the quest for self-knowledge.

Table 3.1 Body Responses/Signals in Stressful Situations

Blushing	Increased heart rate	Breathing changes
Blotching	Know in stomach	Rapid, shallow,
Pallor	Increased peristalsis	deeper, slower
Headache	(stomach rumbling)	Posture changes
Eye squinting	Cramps	Slouching or growing
Teary eyes—welling up	Urinary urgency	smaller
Vision changes	Tightened perineal muscles	Cowering
Dryness of mouth	Leg shakiness	Leaning for support
Grinding teeth	Locked knees, tightened	Leaning toward the other
Clenching teeth	calves Muscle weakness	Turning away
Generalized shakiness	Lump in throat	Crossing arms
Tightness in chest	Changes in voice pitch	Putting hands on hips
Heart pounding	Cold sweat	

This list was adapted from Donnelly G. RN's Survival Sourcebook: Coping With Stress. Oradell, NJ: Medical Economics; 1983.

Appropriate Intimacy

Healthy intimacy with others is a wonderful antidote to unnecessary stress and an effective inoculation against the destructive impact of the · necessary pressures of health care work. Unfortunately, distancing from others or overinvolvement or inappropriate involvement with others can add to our problems in work and at home.

In medical and nursing programs, little is taught on the topic of transference. Transference occurs when a person views someone in the present as if he or she were a significant person from the past. It is a normal phenomenon that we experience often. For instance, when we see a police officer, clergyperson, or someone in authority, we may have a response that has nothing to do with the individual person but has all to do with what they represent to us. Patients and coworkers will often transfer positive and negative feelings onto medical and nursing health care professionals. Being aware of this so as not to absorb the negative transferences or believe and act on the positive ones by violating boundaries is essential.

When one is doing the best that can be done for a patient or is trying to be as supportive as possible to a colleague, it is very hard to recognize negative transference for what it is, but it is important that we do so as not to react negatively in kind. When feeling under great stress at work and/or feeling underappreciated or misunderstood at home, there is also a danger that one would become inappropriately involved with a patient or colleague who is transferring their positive feelings from the past onto us because we are in a caregiving role at a time of great vulnerability and need for them.

Some deal with this not by trying to be aware of what is occurring and discussing it with a trusted senior colleague or mentor but instead by distancing themselves from patients and colleagues alike. Doing this can be dangerous to our welfare and the good of the patients and our colleagues on several levels. First, being very distant can lead to callousness. When this happens, we become impervious to the feelings and needs of others. Also, with respect to our colleagues, deep non-sexual, intimate relationships help one to understand oneself and to open oneself to others in ways that foster mutual support and friendship. In turn, these relationships provide a basis from which we can reach out to patients and colleagues in need.

Learning From Our Negative Emotions

Negative emotions are psychological red lights indicating that we are dealing with situations with which we are unhappy or uncomfortable. It is helpful to more fully understand how contact with people who are depressed, angry, sarcastic, or dismissive of us can affect us. Otherwise, we will respond negatively, passive aggressively, or with "chronic niceness" because of the misguided belief that absorbing patient and colleague anger is part of our job description. As Wicks previously indicated, such an attitude is both dangerous and unnecessary:

> This leads to ulcers, unnecessary stress, depression, and out-bursts of anger when all the "swallowing" of anger becomes too much. Negative emotions are like alcohol; they can be used or abused.
>
> With respect to anger, it needs to be recognized and addressed directly. In addition, if one sees or experiences depression, it too must be named and the source of it questioned. Hiding, belittling, or running away from such emotions because they are unpalatable is only postponing the problem until it gets worse for the other person or the [caregivers] themselves.
>
> Many . . . say: "I just don't know how to deal with angry people." To face such a fear of others' anger or the inexperience one might have in dealing with it, two steps usually are of help to get one started in confronting it.
>
> The first step is imagery. To image oneself dealing with an angry person and to see oneself responding with a sense of poise is a good exercise to practice in the privacy of one's own room. Another useful step when one is holding back from expressing anger in a constructive way is to ask oneself: "What is the worst thing that can happen if I confront someone?"
>
> [Surprisingly more often than you would think] . . . there is a deep fear that the person will beat us up physically. In those instances, I say . . . "If this person is not bigger or tougher than you, it won't happen; if the person is, have someone outside the confrontation area to help you if need be."

We must face our deepest fears about rejection, being
beaten up or having our image stained, so we can face the
blackmail we have set up in our own belief system. This belief
system has been developed over a period and needs to be
addressed so we don't have to continue to run from others'
actual or perceived negative emotions.[17pp254-255]

Through self-questioning, we can arrive at a better recognition of
both direct and indirect expressions of anger. It is also possible through
self-questioning (Box 3.2) that we will see our motivations, fears, and

---

Box 3.2 Questions Regarding Our Experiences of Anger

- In what ways did I make myself angry today? (Not the passive: "What made me angry?")
- With whom did I choose to be angry today? (Once again,
  not the passive: "Who made me angry?")
- As well as the apparent "reason" I was angry, what other
  reasons might there be that I became annoyed, angry, or as
  upset as I was in this particular situation?
- What was my style of dealing with my emotional reaction?
  Did I try to conceal, deny, or play it down?
- How do I normally spontaneously allow my anger to rise
  and come to the surface of my awareness? Did I express
  my anger in a way that was destructive? Was I overly concerned that people would dislike me—even if I expressed
  my anger in a constructive manner?
- Was I able to recognize my anger before it was expressed
  inappropriately ("shotgun fashion" which broadly attacked
  the person and tried to scare him but didn't focus on the
  problem)?
- Did I have a realistic recognition that even good communication around something I am unhappy about may not
  solve the problem? Was I able to take satisfaction in the fact
  that opening a discussion about differences is a worthwhile
  endeavor in itself?

interpersonal style more clearly. The more this is accomplished, the more we will be withdrawing our projections, taking control of our lives, and, in the process, reducing unnecessary stress.

Facing Failure in a Productive Way

A reality in health care is that the more you are involved with persons who are suffering, the more you are going to fail. So, you had better be able to put failure in perspective. There is a myth that if one is up on the literature, pays attention to the patient, and provides an accurate diagnosis and regimen of treatment, failure is impossible. This myth is destructive to the spirit of the medical and nursing professionals. Failure is part and parcel of involvement. And as discussed in Chapter 2, some problems in health care are so "wicked" that failed attempts are common and definitive solutions do not exist. Given the many demands and the inability to be perfectly "on" all the time, failure will occur. People are going to die—unfortunately and occasionally because of our errors or miscalculations. Although this is inevitable when we are constantly dealing with sick people, failure can still provide helpful information that will limit or reframe the approach to future problems. Failure teaches us to

- Recognize the dangers of pride and the need for openness.
- Consider ways to avoid errors in the future.
- Change factors that increase the possibility of failure.
- Learn from failed attempts to change course or strategies.
- Experiment with new approaches.
- Learn about ourselves.
- Improve technique and collaborative style.
- Be sensitive to early warning signs of mistakes.
- Consider the impact of negligence.
- Uncover areas where further education/supervision is required.
- Appreciate unrealistic expectations.
- Improve pacing in one's work.
- Acknowledge personal/professional limitations so they can be corrected or improved and so that we can be more aware of the limitations that will remain unaltered.

- Realize when an attempted solution to a problem becomes the new problem.
- Recognize the unintended consequences of your actions.

If failure is carefully considered rather than just becoming a source of frustration, self-condemnation, or an impetus to blame, deny, or distort the situation, future patients and colleagues will benefit immeasurably from a process of examination on your part. However, to accomplish this, professionals in health care must seek to be critical thinkers.

Critical Thinking

Critical thinking helps us to explore, challenge, and more clearly understand situations, patients and colleagues, as well as our agendas, negative emotions, attitudes, motivations, talents, and growing edges. This not only helps us to have a greater grasp of reality but also stops the drain of psychological energy used up by defensiveness and protecting our image. Because critical thinking is not natural, although we may think it is for us, it takes discipline, a willingness to face the unpleasant, and a stamina that allows one not to become unduly frustrated when we do not achieve results as quickly as we prefer with respect to our insights and growth.

The types of questions we must be willing to ask ourselves as critical thinkers are as follows:

- Am I willing to avoid seeing things simply in black and white?
- Can I entertain diverse viewpoints and be comfortable with ambiguity?
- Can I appreciate that the "answer" or diagnosis I now offer is, at best, tentative?
- When I am discussing a patient, clinical situation, or even my own role, talents, and growing edges as a professional and a person, am I able to entertain both the possible and the probable without undue discomfort?
- Do I need to come to a quick solution or take one side of an issue because I lack the intellectual stamina that encourages an open mind?
- Am I so uncomfortable with personal rejection, a tarnished image, or failure that I capitulate too soon when I disagree with others?

- Am I willing to "unlearn" what I have learned that is no longer useful and be open to new techniques and approaches?
- Do I realize that I resist changes in obvious and less noticeable ways and that one of my goals is to see some of my emotions and extreme reactions as red flags that can often indicate that I may be holding on because of fear, stubbornness, or some other defensive reason?
- Am I willing to engage in a rational debate of the issues, even those I believe to be nonnegotiable or nondebatable?

The willingness to be a critical thinker and face questions like those given not only takes motivation but also involves an appreciation of how resistant most of us usually are without even knowing it.

Appreciating and Overcoming Your Own Resistance to Change

As a French proverb reminds us, the more things change, the more they remain the same. Change—even when we are aware that we have problems that need to be confronted—sometimes seems so elusive. Watzalawick et al.,[18] in the classic work on change, reminds us that to understand change we must consider the value of persistence, of things staying the same, like tradition and dearly held values.

> Whenever change is slow in appearing, common sense suggests that some form of encouragement and perhaps a little push are needed. Similarly, when change does occur, praise and optimism are thought to facilitate more progress. Nothing is usually further from the truth. Incipient change requires a special kind of handling, and the message "Go slow!" is the paradoxical intervention of choice.[19p135]

As Rodman, a psychotherapist, poignantly described, "Every patient stared at long enough, listened to hard enough, yields up a child arrived at from somewhere else, caught up in a confused life, trying to do the right thing, whatever that might be, and doing the wrong thing instead."[20p5] However, Rodman's point does not only hold for persons seeking counseling and psychotherapy. Everyone needs to recognize and explore one's resistances as well, yet even when motivated to do so, this is sometimes easier said than done. It is essential to understand as much as we can about our own hesitancy to both uncover resistances and act effectively to address those areas we need to change. This is especially so if you are a health care professional for whom stress is so intense and working through resistances can literally be the difference between life and death, burnout or not, and living with meaning or drifting in quiet blunted despair.

The concept of resistance in helping patients who are experiencing emotional distress has changed over the years in a way that is helpful for any helping professional wishing to overcome their own barriers to personal and professional growth.

> In the early years of psychology, a client's resistance to change was often looked upon as solely a *motivational* problem. When a person failed in changing, the counselor felt: "I did my job in pointing out your difficulties. In return, you didn't do yours!" The blame rested upon the one seeking change. The goal was to eliminate the resistances and get the person motivated again.
>
> Now, we recognize that when someone resists change and growth in their personal and professional lives, they are not purposely giving family, friends, coworkers, and counselors a hard time. Instead, they are unconsciously providing a great deal of critical information on problematic areas of their life given their personality style, history, and current situation. This material then becomes a real source of new wisdom for psychological growth, professional advancement, and spiritual insight.
>
> Though we still believe motivation is an essential key to making progress, we see that persons seeking change must also gain certain knowledge about themselves and act on it if they wish to advance. Or in a nutshell: *Motivation or positive thinking is good, but it is obviously not enough.*[21p9] (Emphasis is original)

One of the reasons that motivation to change is not a sufficient condition for the alteration of one's attitude, cognition, and behavior is that we fear that the demands of change may be too costly. For instance, we would have to see our own role in the problems we are having and do something about it. In addition, we worry about how other people will react when we seek to move away from defensiveness or unhealthy competitiveness. The move toward health is surprisingly upsetting to those who are used to "the devil they know" with his or her defensive style. It might even challenge them to change, and they would be uncomfortable in dealing with this. Finally, seeing our own role in our problems does cause some negative reflection about the past and how much time we have wasted in behaving as we have. Despite such resistances to insight and growth, though, the "advantages" of staying the same, of persisting as usual, are very costly and the freedom offered by insight and change is very great. In respecting the tyranny of habit and secondary gain, we must take whatever measures we can to make our steps toward self-knowledge and personal/professional growth more realistic. Two ways we can do this is by increasing our sensitivity to our defensiveness and by taking what actions we can to outflank our resistances.

Increasing Sensitivity to Change Resistance—and Outflanking It

When we seek to export the blame for problems in our life, it is referred to as "projection." This defensive style is manifested in many obvious and quiet ways, including denying our role in mistakes or failures, blaming others, excusing our behavior, contextualizing our actions, absolving ourselves, rationalizing failures, and generally removing ourselves from the equation while focusing on the negative roles others have played. Underpinning these actions is that when we try to take responsibility for our own role in various unpalatable events, we go overboard. Instead of trying to understand what part we played so we can learn from this, we move from remorse about what we have done to shame about who we are. We can tell when this occurs because we start to condemn ourselves and become hypercritical of our behavior, overly perfectionistic, unrealistic in our comparison with others in the field, and overresponsible with respect to the impact we did and can have.

Instead, we need to take a step back from the event, to try to frame the situation in an objective way by imagining it was someone else you were observing and to seek to become intrigued about your role. This helps to avoid overly blaming others, condemning yourself, or getting discouraged when results do not happen immediately. To further reduce the resistance to change, the following caveats may work to outflank the blocks to growth:

1. Anything discovered does not have to be changed immediately.
2. No area should be condemned—just neutrally observed as if it were happening to someone else.
3. No area should be defended—no one is criticizing or attacking, just observing where the energy is being spent.
4. Observations—even disturbing ones—should be embraced as a wonderful treasure trove of information.
5. After each period of observation, the areas of concern should be written down, so some record is kept of discovery.[21pp70–71]

With these provisions in mind, we should consider the following principle: "*Where there is energy (positive or negative) there is usually a grasping and/or fear.* When the smoke of a strong reaction is present, the fire of desire is also usually present, and we need to know what it is. Otherwise, rather than our passions being good energy, they may be the product of unexamined attachments"[21p71] (Emphasis is original). Further, our passions then keep us connected to views and convictions that are covering or distorting the truth rather than leading us to it. Classic signs that we are holding on include arguing, not sharing all the information or motivations with persons with whom we discuss the event, complaining that change in certain areas is unrealistic, stonewalling persons through an icy silence or monopolizing the situation, feeling misunderstood or totally ignored, and other strong emotions or off-putting actions.

On the other hand, there are also classic signs that a person does value change, growth, and insight both professionally and personally. Some of these signs are

- An ability to let go.
- Receptivity to new lessons . . .
- Not self-righteous.
- Intrigue with one's own emotional flashing lights.
- Disgust with . . . the endless wheel of suffering that comes from grasping and bad habits.
- Curious, not judgmental.
- Values experience.
- Recognizes danger of preferences which prevent experiencing new gifts in life.
- Awake to present; is mindful.
- Appreciates quiet meditation.
- Generous and alive.

- Learns, reflects, and applies wisdom to daily life.
- Rests lightly in life.[21p78]

In recognizing and overcoming resistances to growth and change, we come to appreciate that the most important person in improving our situation is ourselves. We accept this responsibility not with a spirit of self-condemnation or over-responsibility but with a sense of intrigue about the possibility within ourselves. We acknowledge that at times we are emotional and opinionated. We see that blindness like this occurs because of fear and hesitation, partially rooted in our past and centered in a belief system that is tyrannical and often wrong. This results in a style of self-talk that seems friendly and supportive but in the end undercuts both our ability to see things clearly and develop a level of self-esteem based on knowing what is good about ourselves and what our growing edges are.

Improving Self-Talk

One of the main contributions of cognitive-behavioral psychological theory is its ability to help people better appreciate how one's beliefs (schemata) and cognitions (ways of thinking, perceiving, and understanding) can affect, even drive, feelings and behavior. Unfortunately, dysfunctional ways of perceiving ourselves and the world are both common and often left unchallenged. Such inattention is psychologically dangerous.

Mental health professionals have illustrated how people fall prey to cognitive errors that may lead to depression, an overall sense of discouragement, or both. Perfectionistic medical and nursing professionals can be particularly vulnerable to such irrational thinking patterns. Burns defines the following categories of irrational thinking:

> ALL OR NOTHING THINKING: You see things in black-and-white categories. If your performance falls short of perfect, you see yourself as a total failure . . .
> OVERGENERALIZATION: You see a single negative event as a never-ending pattern of defeat
> MENTAL FILTER: You pick out a single negative detail and dwell on it exclusively so that your vision of all reality becomes

darkened, like the drop of ink that discolors the entire beaker of water

DISQUALIFY THE POSITIVE: You reject positive experiences by insisting that they "don't count" for some reason or other. In this way you can maintain a negative belief that is contradicted by your everyday experiences . . .

EMOTIONAL REASONING: You assume that your negative emotions necessarily reflect the way things are: "I feel it, therefore it must be true . . .

SHOULD STATEMENTS: You try to motivate yourself with should and shouldn't. . . . The emotional consequence is guilt. When you direct "should" statements toward others, you feel anger, frustration, and resentment . . .

PERSONALIZATION: You see yourself as the cause of some negative external event which in fact you were not primarily responsible for.[21pp40–41]

The core of the issue here is as follows:

Negative thinking is quite common. For some reason, all of us seem to give more credence to the negative than to the positive. We can hear numerous positive things but somehow allow a few negative things to discolor and disqualify the previously affirming feedback we received. Therefore, we need to (1) pick up and recognize our negative thinking so we can (2) link the negative thoughts we have to the depressive/anxious feelings we experience, so (3) the negative self-talk we have can be replaced with a more realistic thought or belief. It is in this way that we structure changing our negative thinking so our negative beliefs can eventually be modified as well.

We can always—and unfortunately, frequently do—find a negative comparison to make when we are reflecting on our thoughts, actions, and motivations. . . . Making negative comparisons between our situations and those of others is never a problem. Maintaining perspective . . . is the difficulty!

We may say we already know this but can't seem to put it into practice. When I hear this statement, I think of Mark Twain's comment: "The difference between the right word and the almost right word is the difference between lightning and the lightning bug." We may say we know it, but unless we can truly recognize and short-circuit the negativity that causes insecurity [and] increases defensiveness . . . then we really don't know it.[22pp30-31]

The issue is that the way we perceive something is just as relevant as what we perceive. As the philosopher Epictetus commented in the first century BCE, "What frightens and dismays us is not external events themselves, but the way in which we think about them. It is not things that disturb us, but our interpretation of their significance."[23] When we realize this, then we can see that both successes and failures can be used to increase self-understanding and self-appreciation. This approach is so much more life giving than having our successes and failures be the source of a constant see-saw of ups and downs. When we recognize this, how we look at or question ourselves changes dramatically, as does the overall results.

Questions to Ask in Interviewing Yourself

Self-understanding, not self-indictment, is at the basis of the self-questioning process. This is important to reflect upon again and again—especially when you are conducting a systematic self-evaluation of yourself, your stresses, and the personal and professional goals you have. In addition to having a nonjudgmental attitude when interviewing yourself, a *structured* approach is helpful so that areas are not avoided or missed. When we interview ourselves to uncover cognitive and affectual styles, the chances are great that we may miss or unconsciously avoid some area. Therefore, to aid medical and nursing professionals in the discerning process of improving self-awareness, a Medical/Nursing Professional Secondary Stress Self-Awareness Questionnaire is provided (Box 3.3).

A questionnaire of this type has no right or wrong answers. Although some might find this surprising, there is a tendency to feel awkward or threatened by certain questions even though the question is responded to yourself in confidence. Writing the first thing that comes to mind and trying to be exploratory—rather than judgmental—with yourself will assist in voicing unnecessary defensiveness or the suppression of ideas, thoughts, or feelings we may find uncomfortable.

Box 3.3 Medical/Nursing Professional Secondary Stress
Self-Awareness Questionnaire

Instructions: Find a quiet, comfortable, and private place. Read
each question and respond on a separate sheet of paper by writing the first thing that comes to mind. Once you have completed a page, do not turn back to it or refer to it when working
on succeeding questions. Work as quickly as you can without
setting a pace that is too stressful.

1. What is the reason you believe denial is so prevalent in the
   clinical settings with respect to stress for medical and nursing personnel? What are the most common lies you tell
   yourself about your own stress?
2. At this point, what are the most realistic and helpful steps
   you can take to prevent, limit, and learn from stress?
3. What have you heard are some excellent approaches to
   reducing stress and improving self-care but you feel are
   unrealistic in your case? What would it take to make them
   realistic? ("A miracle!" is not an acceptable answer.)
4. When you think of the terms *burnout, compassion fatigue,* and
   chronic secondary stress, what do you think of in terms of your
   own life?
5. What are the issues that make you most anxious? What are
   the ones you deal with the best?
6. What are the types of situations or interactions from the
   past that still haunt you?
7. Given the realistic demands of work and family, what would
   it take to balance these two areas in your life a bit more?
   (List only those steps that can be realistically taken by you
   within the next 2 to 3 years.)
8. In your own case, what helps you to fall prey to the common masochistic tenet? "The only worthy medical or nursing professional is the one involved enough to be on the
   edge of burnout or physical fatigue."
9. In what ways did your professional schooling, clinical rota-
   tions, modeling by supervisors/teachers, and initial work

after graduation inadvertently teach you that taking care of yourself is a sign of weakness and that an unhealthy lifestyle is the price of being in the field of health care?

10. What are the "bad habits" of the people you observe in your profession that you do not want to emulate? How are you seeking to embrace the wonder, passion, and intense involvement in medicine and nursing without also absorbing the pathological side of the profession?

11. When you are under a great deal of stress, what fantasies do you have? What do you think are healthy fantasies you should act upon some day? What are the unhealthy ones that, if acted upon, would cause you and others harm?

12. What elements that are currently in your self-care protocol have been most beneficial for you? What are the least helpful? Do you have a self-care protocol?

13. What do you struggle with most in your efforts to take care of yourself? Because your presence as a professional in the health care field means that de facto you are a bright and accomplished person, you would not think that these struggles should be so hard for you; why are they?

14. How would people describe your attitudes toward work?

15. What should be included in your list of personal doubts and insecurities that most people would be surprised to know about you?

16. In health care, focus on the person and clinical situation that are before you is essential; what do you find are the main sources of external distraction and inner preoccupation that prevent you from doing this?

17. What are the most positive and negative affects your personality style exhibits in the way you interact with patients? With staff?

18. When under extreme stress, what is your style of interacting with others and handling the situation that you would most like to change? What steps are necessary to produce such a change?

19. What would you include in your list of motivations for originally becoming a medical or nursing professional? (Make the list as long as you can. Be sure to include any reasons you might now perceive as unrealistic or possibly immature—e.g., status, power over other people's life and death struggles, financial security, voyeurism, etc.—so you have as complete an accounting as possible.)

20. Has the primacy of certain motivations changed for you over time? If so, how? Why do you think this is so? If this is problematic in some way, what might you do about it? For those beneficial changes in priorities, how are you ensuring that they remain in focus for you?

21. What are the most awkward subjects for you to discuss in relationship to your emotional and physical well-being as a health professional?

22. Where do you feel your narcissism comes into play in your role in health care?

23. What would be included in a list of what you like best about being a medical or nursing professional? What would be on the list of what you like least?

24. What is most surprising to you about the professional life you now have?

25. What are the most frustrating aspects of your professional life? Your personal life?

26. If you have ever considered changing specialties, moving to a different health care setting, or leaving the field, what are the reasons for this?

27. When you think of the profession you are now a part of, how would you describe it for someone thinking of entering the field now? Suppose someone asked you how you thought it would be different in 5 years, what would you say?

28. What are the most important self-care procedures you have put into place in the past 5 years? What has been their impact on you? What ways would you now like to modify your plan?

29. Given your own personality style, what types of patients do you find most challenging? What types of colleagues, subordinates, and supervisors can easily elicit an emotional reaction from you? Given this, what ways have you found to effectively interact with them? (Praying for their early happy death is not a sufficient response.)

30. How would you describe the seemingly beneficial and adverse impacts your professional life has had on your personal life and vice versa?

31. What are the 5 mistakes that you fear most in your work?

32. What stresses do you think you can lessen in your life by giving them some attention? What stresses do you feel powerless to alter?

33. How would you describe the differences in the sources of stress and the approaches to self-care between other human services fields and that of medicine and nursing?

34. How self-aware do you feel you are? On what do you base this conclusion? What would help you gain greater self-awareness?

35. If you were to divide your personal needs for happiness into "necessary" and "desirable," what would be on each list? What would be on similar lists ("necessary" and "desirable") for professional satisfaction and growth?

36. What information about yourself do you think you are most likely to hide even from yourself because it makes you uncomfortable to be aware of it?

37. What is your style of dealing with conflict? How would you improve your approach? To accomplish this, what is the next step you think you should take?

38. How much time alone do you need to remain balanced? What are the means you use to enable that such time is scheduled for yourself?

39. How do you know when you have lost your sense of perspective? What steps do you take to regain or maintain it?

40. What role does a sense of humor and laughter play in keeping yourself and the situation you are in from getting unnecessarily "heavy?"

41. What "little things" in life do you treasure and would miss if they were not present in your life? What are the "big things? How do you show that you appreciate them?

42. Of what professional accomplishments are you very proud? What are some future ones you would very much like to achieve?

43. Describe how you organize your schedule and how much control you have in your life? Are there ways this might be improved?

44. When and with whom are you most apt to react in an angry way? In a cowardly way? By withdrawing? Through avoidance?

45. Would you and others at work and home best describe you as assertive, passive, passive-aggressive, or aggressive? Is there a difference between your style in your personal life and that in your professional life? If so, how do you account for that?

46. What are the major areas of imbalance in your life? How are you addressing them? If you are not, what are some of the reasons you feel it is important to do so at this point in your life?

47. Do you know how to observe your feelings and behavior and then seek to see what cognitions (ways of thinking, perceiving, and understanding) and beliefs (schemata) are giving rise to them? If so, do you then dispute your dysfunctional thoughts in an attempt to keep perspective and avoid unnecessary stress/depressive thinking/self-condemnation? If not, how might you improve this area of self-awareness, self-monitoring, and increased recognition of the style of one's self-talk, especially when under undue stress or after a failure?

48. What are the unhealthiest ways you are now meeting your needs or "medicating" yourself? What unhealthy

gratifications are you concerned that you might avail your-self of in the future? What are you doing to prevent, limit, or avoid this from happening?

49. What is the overall design of your daily, weekly, monthly, and yearly breaks for leisure, relaxation, quiet, and recreation? How would you describe your feelings about these times (e.g., guilt, "I deserve it," feeling uncomfortable, preoccupied with cases, blissful, resentment that they are too few and far between, etc.)?

50. What are the types of negative statements you normally make to yourself when you fail?

51. What are the healthiest ways you cope with life's difficulties? What are the most immature and unhealthy ways?

52. In what ways are you collaborative with other members of the health care team? What are the benefits and struggles you experience with such collaboration?

53. What professional and personal resentments do you still carry, and when are they most likely to surface?

54. Have you had any significant losses in the past several years? If so, what has your reaction been to them—initially, recently, now?

55. How do you view yourself in terms of physical aspects of your life (e.g., attractiveness, physical health, eating/drinking/weight/smoking/medication and illegal drug use, and exercise patterns)?

56. What is your reaction to the statement, "Much of medical care is still an art rather than an exact science"?

57. What are your feelings about asking for help in your personal life from your family? A colleague? Professional organization? One's physician? A psychiatrist, psychologist, or counselor? A clergyperson?

58. In your professional life, have you been tempted to step over personal, sexual, financial, or other appropriate boundaries you should have with your patients or colleagues?

59. Is there someone in your circle of friends who is kind yet clear and direct with you, so you would feel at ease to

share anything but also would feel you are getting honest guidance?

60. In what clinical situations or with what type of clients do you feel most emotionally vulnerable? In other words, when have you reacted by going to either the extreme of overinvolvement or preoccupation or by closing down emotionally and seeing them as simply "a case," "bed 2 in room 342," or "the gallbladder in intensive care"?

Permission to reprint this form can be gained without cost by indicating copyright (© 2005 Robert J. Wicks) and source (R. Wicks, *Overcoming Secondary Stress in Medical and Nursing Practice*, New York: Oxford University Press; 2020) and sending a written request indicating the reason and audience for its intended use to Dr. Robert J. Wicks, E-mail: rwicks@loyola.edu.

If a questionnaire of this type can elicit an almost matter-of-fact style of answering, it will provide a wonderful resource of information on how we are thinking, feeling, and acting in our professional and personal lives. The combination of answers can also provide themes that offer a springboard to real understanding and insight into our personalities. Of course, on the other hand, those individuals who are defensive and try to coach their answers or are vague will end up with little helpful material other than the conclusion that how they look to themselves without reflection is the same, even after time is spent reviewing intrapersonal and interpersonal styles, talents, growing edges, and personal/professional hopes and goals.

In addition to acting as a guide to quiet reflection by yourself, the responses to the questionnaire can be helpful in speaking with a mentor, trusted family member or coworker, or counselor or as material for a discussion group. Another value in its use is that it provides a record for us. By having in writing a clear description of our thoughts and feelings about key areas in our lives, we can go back to them again and again to see how they match our current outlook. Moreover, once we have our original impressions down on paper, our unconscious censoring mind cannot change what we have written, and our memory cannot distort our impressions as easily. A final advantage in this personal process is that by reviewing previously noted reactions, we can discover what additional thoughts we now have about such issues, thus tapping into our personal wisdom and expanding upon it.

As in any challenging undertaking, there are resistances to taking the time to accomplish the task at hand. Yet, if someone early in your education told you that you would improve your chances significantly, to be accepted into a professional school, by taking only an hour or so of your time to complete a questionnaire, you would probably jump at it. The same can be said of completing this questionnaire with respect to the remaining years of your professional career. By taking time to focus on yourself in a helpful, guided way, there is immeasurable aggravation you can avoid and pleasure, control, and balance in your life you can more fully enjoy.

Reviewing Your Responses

Once you have completed the questionnaire, it may be helpful in your reflective process and in discussion of the topics with trusted others to have a guide. However, even before you consider a series of suggestions on what a question might elicit in terms of responses, it is important to take great caution in considering what you have written. Interpretations or attempts to deeply understand your responses should always be viewed as tentative. Even the most experienced mental health specialists can make incorrect or partially correct interpretations or explanations of individual responses. Therefore, the Medical/Nursing Professional Secondary Stress Self-Awareness Questionnaire is intended as a springboard for further reflection on your part or discussion with someone else as to what your response might mean with respect to implications for self-care, self-knowledge, or the prevention or limitation of secondary stress in your life. *Remember:* The knowledge provided by your responses to the questionnaire will facilitate an even better understanding than you now have of your lifestyle patterns, talents, and growing edges. The questionnaire is not an exercise in guilt enhancement or a means to increase your narcissism. Your attitude toward the review will be the major factor in gleaning valuable information from it. In reviewing what you have written, there are two final points to consider:

1. Before beginning the review, try to set the stage for a non-judgmental review of the material by assuming a sense of intrigue rather than defensive projection, self-condemnation, or discouragement. One way to accomplish this is to imagine that you are looking at the profile of someone else rather than yourself. Such an artificial distancing from the material might help in limiting judgmental or unduly defensive tendencies.

2. Read each response to each question and think about the meaning of what you have written. The pace of this process will be different for each individual. Sometimes we spend a good deal of time on a particular response that touches a personal chord in our lives at the time. Other times, the area being questioned has little emotional weight or application at this time in your life.

Having offered these provisos, a listing of *some* factors that may be helpful to consider in reflecting on your responses to each of the questions is provided (Box 3.4). Just use them as a catalyst to your own ideas. In this way, you will make the evaluation of the questionnaire your own and, with greater self-knowledge, be more apt to follow through on what you think are the logical, realistic self-care steps you might develop after reviewing the final chapters in this book.

Self-knowledge and self-care have taken on new urgency as a function of our experiences with the COVID-19 pandemic. We do not yet know the full effects of living through the pandemic on medical and nursing professionals themselves nor on the future of the health professions. Will the pandemic promote the enactment of self-care protocols by medical and nursing professionals? Will the pandemic ignite the "passion to care" in future generations or not? Will the professions be able to recruit committed and caring individuals? Will the health care system successfully retain and nurture those medical and nursing professionals that worked so tirelessly under difficult conditions to care for those infected? Will we feel more isolated or more connected to community postpandemic?

In the personal quest for self-awareness and life perspective, particularly, considering the recent pandemic, it is well to remember:

A healthy perspective does not deny the tough times in life. Instead, it allows us to face them directly with the understanding that it is not the amount of darkness in the world or even

Box 3.4 Reflection Guide for Each Question in the Medical/
Nursing Professional Secondary Stress Self-Awareness
Questionnaire in Box 3.3.

1. We often tell ourselves "lies" about our behavior and make
   excuses for it because we do not want to give up the
   secondary gain involved or expend the effort needed to
   decrease the amount of stress we are experiencing. Until
   the "payoffs" we receive for the behavior are unmasked
   as too costly and unnecessary, even the most destructive
   and immature defensive behavior will continue to cause us
   stress.

2. "Realistic" and "helpful" are important words in this question because they try to help us get around the resistance
   to change that is present when we feel that any steps to
   reduce stress in health care are beyond us; therefore, we do
   not have to do anything.

3. This question seeks to push us a bit further to get us to
   be more assertive and creative in our planning and actions
   regarding the stress in life.

4. Too often we resist change by being global in our definitions of what is causing stress in our lives. This question
   seeks to get more specific causes out in the open so they
   can be addressed more directly either by ourselves or with
   our mentor/peer group.

5. This question allows us to make an inventory of our
   strengths and areas of vulnerability or growing edges. The
   longer and more detailed the two lists, the more useful will
   be the responses. Also, looking for patterns in the list can
   be helpful in terms of planning interventions or attitude/
   schedule changes.

6. The only memory that is a problem is the one intentionally forgotten or unconsciously repressed because it retains
   power without our being aware of it. This question gives an
   opportunity to be honest again regarding those past events
   that are still sapping energy from us now and unconsciously

impacting our behaviors in the present. PTSD includes such memories, but anyone who works in health care, by nature of their work, has experienced traumatic occurrences and needs to have a clear awareness of them—not in order to blame oneself but to learn from them.

7. In health care, there is a general tendency toward an imbalance in favor of work over one's personal life. This question provides an opportunity to take initial steps to change this imbalance a bit. One of the goals in phrasing the question again with the word "realistic" is to try to break the logjam that occurs when we feel overwhelmed and think nothing can be done. Perspective and attitude have tremendous power; although people who burn out often lose an awareness of this and feel that unless someone else changes my environment, little of benefit can result.

8. Once we accept the mantle of "only a burned out professional really cares and works hard," the psychological cost is immense. Moving against this societal and professional myth is essential if one is to undertake a program of self-care.

9. This is an opportunity to divide the people who we thought were professionally competent and personally attractive from the dysfunctional behavior they may have also modeled.

10. As a follow-up to question 9, this one asks for more information on how we can carry on the good heritage of our role models and leave their parallel defensive sides so we can become more healthy in how we carry out medical/ nursing roles.

11. There are some fantasies we should act on and others that would be dangerous if we did. Knowing the difference ahead of time is essential, so acting out or violating boundaries with colleagues or patients is never done with the rationalization after the fact that "It just happened."

12. This raises the need to have a self-care protocol and starts us thinking in a more-focused manner about the helpful

and destructive ways one deals with the pressures in one's personal and professional life.

13. This question is designed to have one face their own resistances and defenses with the same energy and intellectual stamina as other issues are faced in life.

14. "Workaholism" is a pattern that seems to go unchecked in many a health care professional's life; this question helps one not to gloss over the work style that everyone seems to acknowledge is present in us but that we cannot seem to fully grasp ourselves. People continue to endure an immense amount of unnecessary stress with either the response "It's part of the territory . . . this is what we signed up for . . . as a medical or nursing professional" or "That's just the way I am."

15. This allows us to take a step back and to acknowledge the human doubts and insecurities that all people have. This is important because much defensive or compensatory behavior is driven by such unexamined dynamics.

16. Distractions waste a tremendous amount of time in health care. Mistakes are often attributed to a lack of attention. This question helps us to see how we might systemically avoid unnecessary distraction or understand the dynamics involved in what needlessly preoccupies us when at work.

17. Making a list of how our personality both negatively and positively affects certain types of individuals when we are in certain moods, equips us to better use our style of dealing with the world. By having greater awareness in this area, we can avoid so many potential relational problems. It is worth returning to this question to see what else we might add as illustrations of when and how we improved or made situations worse. It is difficult to do this because of the tendency to project the blame onto a patient or staff member on the one hand or simply blame ourselves on the other. Clarity and a non-judgmental approach to ourselves and our behavior are needed here.

18. Knowing your own stress points and when you are particularly vulnerable is essential. Even basic steps like knowing when to keep quiet until we understand why we are reacting so strongly and can regain more of our composure can make a major difference in the stress level of interactions with others.

19. In many cases we believe we know why we entered the field of medicine or nursing. However, there were many overlapping mature and immature reasons that we probably have not thought about. Having this information is very valuable so that we can appreciate how to let the mature reasons grow and the other ones atrophy or take their proper place rather than ascending to a level where we make decisions for the wrong reasons.

20. Revisiting motivations that inspired and challenged us is essential if we are to keep and deepen the roles we have assumed in the lives of others. This reflection is very important, in light of the jaded views of many in the culture with respect to health care and the possible beneficial roles they might play in it.

21. There are many awkward subjects that are sensitive for us to discuss with others that we do not reflect on "in safety" with ourselves. This question gives us permission and encouragement to take the time to examine what we are sensitive about and to ask ourselves what we can do about it.

22. Healthy narcissism is good. It encourages us to take credit for good work and to be happy that we are in key roles caring for others. It also helps us recognize when we become defensive because our ego is getting in the way when it should not.

23. This question reacquaints us with both the joy and pain of being in health care. It is asked so that there is greater clarity about what we do not like to see and how it can be changed in some way; even minor alterations in a number of areas can provide great summative relief. But more than

that, by getting clearer about what we like best, we can remember to enjoy and take strength from these areas as they are encountered each day.

24. This is a standard "taking stock" question that asks us what is going on that we did not anticipate. Therefore, if we need to do something about it we can do it before we become too derailed personally and professionally.

25. Frustrations drain energy. By naming them we are taking the first step to understanding why they are so frustrating to us whereas others do not find them to be so. Once they can be understood in this way, they will lose some of their power; then we can catch ourselves when we repeat the pattern.

26. Thoughts of job change often come at times when we have an aggregate of negative elements in our professional lives. By reviewing when and how we thought of moving on or actually did, we can learn ways that may prevent unnecessary moves, We can also realize more fully when such a significant change is needed to relieve intractable stress or open up new possibilities.

27. This question is important for all of us to ask. It encourages us to be honest with ourselves concerning how we feel about the field we have chosen and our role in it. It also pulls us into the future to give some sense of the tone of our outlook, and it begs the question, "What would I need to do to make this more positive for myself?"

28. Our self-care protocol is examined here. At the very least, this question will encourage us to see if we have a plan in place. If it is informal, then it will help us write down what we are doing and give us a sense of how we might improve it.

29. Knowing who "pushes our emotional buttons" is an important antidote to unnecessary stress. This question revisits this area so that greater clarity, which is much needed if we are to remain psychologically healthy in tense situations, can be gained. Otherwise, the only thing that will happen

is that we will project blame onto certain types of people or blame ourselves for losing our temper or acting out.

30. Looking at the interchange between personal and professional well-being and how they affect each other helps us see that most adversity involves a more complex dynamic than we first imagined.

31. Breaking down fear into specifics allows us to discuss the elements with mentors and colleagues whom we trust. This leads to dealing with fears constructively rather than having them haunt us to no purpose. Just a naming and discussion of these fears can help alleviate stress in this area.

32. Powerlessness is an element in all of us. However, once again, perception and attention to such areas tend to diminish those factors that heretofore have been ignored and allowed to take control as a function of a lack of examination.

33. This is a chance to see what, if any, differences we feel about our profession and the stresses it holds as opposed to other fields. It allows us also to normalize some of our stress because we have much in common with persons in many fields but do not often acknowledge this.

34. Methods that lead to self-awareness such as reflection, meditation, journaling, receiving and giving supervision, personal daily debriefing, receiving mentoring, and formal/informal peer group discussions can help us become better attuned to our styles. This question helps us visit this area to see if any of these approaches are present in some way, and if not, why not.

35. By breaking down needs, we can discern those cases where we are depriving ourselves of essential needs for personal or professional well-being and where we have developed a series of induced needs that are psychologically costing us too much.

36. This question again visits the issue of shame. It allows us to free up those areas we have partially hidden even from ourselves so we can finally learn more from them and let

them take a more appropriate place in our psyche rather than dominating from within.

37. Each person has a different style of dealing with conflict. It is neither good nor bad; it just "is." By taking this approach and considering the pros and cons of our style, we can take steps to improve upon it. Most people focus on whether the other person is right or wrong rather than on the style of conflict resolution. That is why this question, if responded to in detail, can be very fruitful and can be a significant factor in stress reduction for ourselves and for those with whom we interact.

38. Time alone is often considered a luxury or seems to just happen at times in our schedule. However, whether you are an introvert or an extrovert, time alone is psychologically needed for renewal, reflection, and reassessment and to break the movement of an often-driven schedule. Having greater intention on where, how, and when to insert periods of solitude is necessary for one's mental health and for those who are religiously minded is an element of most major spiritualities.

39. Our loss of perspective is often more evident to others than to ourselves. However, there are signs that we have lost distance and a sense of proportion. They include extreme emotion, withdrawal, an unnecessary increase in the pace of activity, and preoccupation. Once we know this, we can then ask ourselves how to best regain perspective. It may be by taking a few minutes alone on a short walk around the hospital or retreating to the staff lounge, a telephone call to a friend, or just remaining silent until we regain more of our composure. This approach helps us realize that each day we lose perspective and need to regain it in some way. It also prevents the three classic dangers that come about when perspective is lost: projection, self-blame, and discouragement. Intrigue with the dynamics within us and within the context in which the loss of perspective occurred is healthy

and productive. Answering this question fully helps support positive movement in our professional and personal lives.

40. Too often, on the way to taking our work seriously, we take ourselves too seriously. This question highlights this reality for all of us and helps us remember to continually appreciate that laughter is good medicine, especially laughing at ourselves, and a sense of humor lightens one's perspective.

41. Deep gratitude is one of the major preventatives and antidotes to a loss of perspective. We have much to be grateful for—including our roles in health care, which not everyone can or is willing to undertake. Gratitude is not natural for most of us, whereas negative reactions seem to rise spontaneously and without effort. Self-training in this area, starting with greater awareness that all is a gift, can provide an immeasurable factor in the prevention of burnout. This is so because when you are feeling constantly nourished by your surroundings, you retain a better sense of balance— gratitude increases our sensitivity to what events and people are giving us so we do not take them for granted, belittle them, or in fact miss them.

42. Taking stock of your accomplishments is an act of healthy narcissism. It also aids, once again, in prevention of the loss of perspective that comes when we just focus on the failures, absences, and struggles without seeing how far we have come. It also aids in planning for the future, which stirs up new hope in our hearts rather than having us just go through the motions every day.

43. Time management is often not taught to medical and nursing professionals. Yet, one of the causes of stress is disorganization or distraction at work. This question raises this issue to imply that there is more in our control than we are willing to acknowledge. In developing a self-care protocol, this area must be addressed in some way so we can use management/organizational skills to lessen stress. (This is addressed in Chapter 5 on developing a self-care protocol.

44. By picturing actual people in our lives who cause attack-or-flight reactions, we can better understand what this type of person is triggering in our lives and so better deal with it. Once again, in most people's lives, the fact that certain people or personality types upset us is accepted as a given that cannot be changed. In medicine and nursing, this is a luxury of avoidance that must not be accepted, because we need to deal with such persons again and again.

45. Appreciating our style by honestly looking at ourselves should be easier at this point in the questionnaire because by now, we should be into the exercise of looking with a sense of intrigue and not with condemnation or denial. As we do this, it is important to see the differences in our styles at work and at home and try to better understand them. This will help in improving our interaction skills both at home and in our health care work setting.

46. Imbalances need not remain in our lives. They also need not be radically corrected overnight. Such a desire often ends up in our acting rashly rather than courageously to provide the necessary balance that will result in personal and professional well-being.

47. Picking up on our feelings about things and then looking at what we are thinking and believing that may be dys-functional and responding to them with thoughts that are healthier are important steps in maintaining perspective and mental health. This question highlights this process and helps to raise the volume of our "self-talk" so we do not let negative thinking act as the invisible puppeteer in our psyche.

48. Work-a-holism, alcohol abuse, improper use of medication, sexual acting out, and compulsive activity (eating, buying, or gambling/stock market speculation) are just a few ways in which we "self-medicate." Knowing how, when, and to what extent we do this is an important first step in address-ing this problematic area and is often one of the important steps that we deny.

49. Taking time off during the day, week, month, and year is a conscious decision by those who effectively prevent and limit burnout. This area, as well as our feelings about them, is important to address as part of self-care.

50. Failure is part and parcel of involvement. The more we are involved and the more delicate problems we must face in health care, the more we will fail. This is a statistical reality because we cannot be perfect. Case closed. Therefore, knowing how we deal with failure, because it is a part of what we do, would help diminish unnecessary anxiety and avoidable stress.

51. This question addresses overall style when we are faced with obstacles. It also asks for an inventory of our talents and defenses. As in some of the other questions, this seeks a review and goes hand in hand with other questions to check the reliability of our previous responses.

52. Collaboration is often seen as necessary but not realistic by many in health care. Yet, to be effective, health care needs to be a team effort in which each member of the team is respected, given as much autonomy as is appropriate, and has input into the health care program offered for the patient. An individual's understanding and attitude toward collaboration are explored in this question.

53. Resentments are psychological powder kegs that lie in the preconscious and may break through when triggered by an event or a person in our environment—especially when sleep deprivation or another problem/lack is present to make us more vulnerable. Unearthing these resentments so they do not remain as hidden psychological cancers that go unnoticed but continue to grow and devour us from within is obviously necessary.

54. Because dealing with the issues of death and dying is part of the territory for health care professionals, being aware of our own losses and how we have dealt with them or avoided dealing with them is quite helpful.

55. Taking note of our physical prowess and those elements that add or are destructive to it is something that is paradoxically avoided by many in health care. This question asks for a detailed response that is undertaken without blame but with honesty and a willingness to consider measured change that will not be abandoned as in the case of a diet that leaves us permanently deprived.

56. Not every error in medical and nursing care is malpractice. No medical or nursing professional can be perfect in their diagnosis or intervention with all patients. This is a reality of the fact that neither medicine nor nursing is perfect. How we answer this question provides some insight into our view of the expectations we have of ourselves and the field.

57. We can never go it alone. Also, sometimes it is important to treat ourselves to a defined period of therapy or mentoring so we can work through failures, deepen our personal lives, and learn new creative ways of improving personal and professional well-being. This question looks at how we avail ourselves of help, collaboration, supervision, and support.

58. Honesty in this question allows us to pick up the "emotional flags" that will warn us when we might violate boundaries with a patient or colleague. Everyone has a vulnerable place in their lives where boundary violation is possible. Knowing ahead of time what these may be or what type of person with whom we would be most vulnerable is essential.

59. This question identifies those with whom we feel both freedom and clarity. At the very least, posing this question points to the tenet that if we do not have a person like this, we run the risk of going off course in our professional and personal lives. It also points to the need to ensure we have steady contact with someone like this and, if we do not, to find someone who can fit this role.

60. Becoming callous or overemotional is a constant danger in health care. This question is designed to help us explore

when and how this happens. As in the other questions in this questionnaire, it is asking us not to take our reactions for granted but to explore them further so we can both understand ourselves better and plan for change that is productive both professionally and personally.

in ourselves that matters, it is how we stand in that darkness that is crucial.[24p51]

References

1. Southgate L. Foreword. In: Salinsky J, Sacklin P, eds., *What Are You Feeling, Doctor?* Oxford, UK: Radcliffe Medical Press; 2000: viii.
2. Baker E. *Caring for Ourselves.* Washington, DC: American Psychiatric Association; 2003.
3. Coster J, Schwebel M. Well-functioning in professional psychologists. *Professional Psychology: Research and Practice.* 1997;28:10.
4. Block D. Foreword. In: Schott C, Hawk J, eds. *Heal Thyself.* New York, NY: Brunner/Mazel; 1986: ix.
5. Wicks R. *Touching the Holy.* Notre Dame, IN: AMP; 1992.
6. Chadwick D. *The Crooked Cucumber.* New York, NY: Broadway; 1999.
7. De Chant P, Shannon DW. *Preventing Physician Burnout: A Handbook for Physicians and Health Care Leaders.* North Charleston, SC: Simpler Healthcare; 2016.
8. Brazier D. *Zen Therapy.* New York, NY: Wiley; 1995.
9. Wicks R. *Availability.* New York, NY: Crossroad; 1986.
10. e.e. cummings. Unpublished letter to a high school editor, 1955. From the October 26th, 1955 edition of the Ottawa Hills High School Spectator (Grand Rapids, Michigan).
11. Pfifferling, JH. Cultural antecedents promoting professional impairment. In: Scott C, Hawk J, eds. *Heal Thyself.* New York, NY: Brunner/Mazel; 1986.
12. Coombs R, Fawzy F. The impaired-physician syndrome: a developmental perspective. In: Scott C, Hawk J, eds. *Heal Thyself.* New York, NY: Brunner/Mazel, 1986.
13. Auden WH. Introduction. In: Hammarskjold D, *Markings.* New York: Knopf; 1976: ix.

14. Leech K. *Soul Friend*. San Francisco, CA: Harper and Row; 1980.
15. Aitken R. *The Mind of Clover: Essays on Zen Buddhist Ethics*. San Francisco, CA: North Point Press; 1984.
16. Hanh TH. *No Mud, No Lotus: The Art of Transforming Suffering*. Berkeley, CA: Parallax Press; 2014.
17. Wicks R. The stress of spiritual ministry: practical suggestions on avoiding unnecessary distress. In: Wicks R, ed. *Handbook of Spirituality for Ministers*. Vol. 1. Mahwah, NJ: Paulist Press; 1995: 254–255.
18. Watzalawick P, Weakland J, Fisch R. *Change: Principles of Problem Formation and Problem Resolution*. New York, NY: W. W. Norton; 1974.
19. Rodman R. *Keeping Hope Alive*. New York, NY: Harper and Row; 1985.
20. Wicks, R. *Simple Changes*. Notre Dame, IN: Thomas More/Sorin Books; 2000.
21. Burns D. *Feeling Good*. New York, NY: New American Library; 1980.
22. Wicks R. *Living Simply in an Anxious World*. Mahwah, NJ: Paulist Press; 1988.
23. Epictetus. *The Art of Living: The Classical Manual on Virtue, Happiness and Effectiveness*. Lebell S, ed. New York, NY: Harper One, 1994.
24. Wicks R. Resilience in a time of crisis. *Nursing* 2020;50(6):49–51.

FOUR

Drawing from the Well of Wisdom

Three Core Spiritual Approaches to Maintaining Perspective and Strengthening the Inner Life of the Medical and Nursing Professionals

Objectives

- Define the role of the inner life in the amelioration of stress.
- Consider the value and challenges of silence and solitude in overcoming stress.
- Explore the benefits of meditation.
- Identify the power of humor in strengthening the inner life and human connection.
- Consider the benefits of friendship and community.
- Evaluate one's ability to listen and reflect.

> *The cyclone derives its powers from a calm center. So does a person.*
> —Dominic of Calaruega

My mother, in the end stages of dementia, received in-home hospice care for 5 months. I made it a point to be there every Friday morning when our hospice nurse, Moira, made her weekly visit. I would ask her questions about the dying process, what I should look for and how I could make Mom more comfortable. On one occasion I explained to Moira that Mom seemed very restless and the morphine was not doing much good. "What was your Mom's favorite music when she was young?" Moira asked. I showed Moira a picture of my mother in

*her 1920's flapper costume and recounted how much Mom loved the
"Charleston," her favorite dance. The following week, Moira brought
a tape of Charleston dance selections that I played when Mom seemed
agitated. It worked—in fact, every now and then Mom would faintly
smile amidst her new calm."*

*Moira was born and raised in Ireland where she attended nursing
school before emigrating to the US. She and I compared notes about
our work in nursing. She shared many funny stories about working in
hospice nursing which I found surprising. She was so good at caring
for the dying, a part of nursing from which I had purposely distanced.
Moira helped me understand the dying process and taught me the
signs of impending death. She accurately predicted the week of my
Mother's death. She attended my Mom's funeral where I finally got
the courage to ask, "How do you deal with the stress of death and
dying every day? How does it not drive you to despair?" I will never
forget her response, in that deep Irish accent, "Every mornin' before
I go to work, I sit in my favorite chair, close my eyes and say a prayer.
Then, I open the daily newspaper to the 'Irish Sports Page' and read
every listing." "What is the Irish sports page?" I asked. "It's the
obituary pages, my dear. It helps to know that we will all be listed
there someday"*

Medical and nursing professionals cannot avoid stress, but its effects
do not have to be totally negative. Moira's approach to hospice work
illustrates that even amid the suffering, maybe even *because* of it, one's
appreciation of life's meaning and all it holds may become even deeper,
enhancing our compassion.

How medical and nursing professionals *perceive* their work, the
events that take place in the course of a day, and the people they
encounter along the way make all the difference. Due to this, an
increasing number of health care professionals are turning to aspects
of the wisdom literature of the major religions as a resource to maintain a sense of psychological perspective. In addition, research and
publications confirming the spirituality/religion (R/S) and health
dynamic have grown exponentially in recent years. These publications
explore the R/S—health connection of patients, significant others,
and clinicians.

In a systematic review of 3000 articles published from 1872 to 2010,
Koenig,[1pp1-3] examined the relationship between R/S and health. This

analysis yielded specific clinical implications with respect to spirituality and care:

- Patients' spiritual needs, related to medical and psychiatric illnesses, often go unmet especially those associated with terminal illnesses. Unmet spiritual needs can adversely affect health.
- A large percentage of patients use R/S to cope with their illnesses and for many R/S is their main coping mechanism.
- Patients' R/S beliefs influence their medical decisions and can enhance or interfere with compliance to those treatments.
- Medical decisions made by physicians are often influenced by their own R/S beliefs particularly with respect to the use of pain medications, abortion, vaccinations, and contraception, but physician beliefs are not discussed with patients.
- Since R/S is correlated with both mental and physical health, health professionals need information about how such influences work.
- The kind of care and support that patients receive when discharged is often shaped by the R/S family or community of faith.
- The standards set by hospital accrediting bodies and government organizations such as the Center for Medicare Services require that medical and nursing professionals respect patients' values and beliefs including R/S.

Koenig concludes that the combination of R/S and health has moved into the mainstream of health care. It is therefore necessary for medical and nursing professionals to have knowledge about the interface between R/S and health to enhance not only patient care but self-care as well.

Pargament, a respected researcher in this area, points out that "every religion offers a set of cognitive reframing mechanisms to help individuals conserve a sense of meaning in life in the face of what may seem to be senseless, unbearable or unjust."[2] According to Hood et al.[3] religion also helps people regain a sense of control that helps them cope and adjust when they are faced with difficult situations. Herbert Benson,[4] a cardiologist, studied the practices of world religious and secular groups. He found that nearly every human civilization employed practices, often religiously oriented, to quiet the mind and relax the body. He studied the effects of these practices on physiological parameters. He coined the term "relaxation response" to describe the physiological changes he observed, such as decreases in respiratory rate, heart rate, and metabolism during states of relaxation. Benson's research is now focusing on the long-term results of practicing meditative/relaxation techniques. The mind–body effects of these practices include the activation of genes that control metabolism, stress, and the aging of the body and the quieting of genes that control the body's immune system.[5]

Despite the mounting evidence, there remains a caution or, at the very least, a hesitancy about discussing where this fits in the life of medical and nursing professionals. This is understandable if we speak of religion with its canons; this is a very private area in everyone's life. Johnston-Taylor[6] asserts that in the last few decades, concurrent with societal trends, nurses have embraced the concept of spirituality while avoiding discussions of religion, even though spirituality can be considered the personal aspect of religious experience. Johnston-Taylor's book, *Fast Facts About Religion for Nurses: Implications for Patient Care*,[6] lists the basic tenets of major religions and the clinical implications of such beliefs so that the nurse can interact more effectively with patients, always respecting the patient's beliefs.

Beyond religion, with all that it offers some people, there is the broad sense of spirituality or faith that is an outgrowth of one's beliefs about life. This can have an impact not only on how we process potentially stressful events but also on how we interact with patients. For our purposes here, we mean "faith" in the broadest sense of the term.

The Sanskrit word for *faith* is *visvas*, which literally translated means "to have trust, to breathe freely, to be without fear." Being able to offer yourself, your colleagues, and your patients' encounters marked by such psychological space can make all the difference. It is irrelevant whether we say that the approach is based on our faith, attitude, outlook, or the more inclusive term *inner life*.

The inner life or interior life is what spiritual figures point to as a place where ego strength, simplicity, freedom, and truth flourish. It is the place in which deeply felt needs are experienced and addressed; these include

A need for permanence in a civilization of transience.
A need for the Absolute when all else is becoming relative.
A need for silence amid noise.
A need for generosity in the face of unbelievable greed.
A need for poverty amid the flaunting of wealth.

A need for contemplation in a century of action, for without contemplation, action risks becoming mere agitation.

A need for communication in a universe content with entertainment and sensationalism.

A need for peace amid today's universal outbursts of violence.

A need for quality to counterbalance the increasingly prevalent response to quantity.

A need for humility to counteract the arrogance of power and science.

A need for human warmth when everything is being rationalized or computerized.

A need to belong to a small group rather than to be part of the crowd.

A need for slowness to compensate the present eagerness for speed.

A need for truth when the real meaning of words is distorted in political speeches and sometimes even in religious discourses.

A need for transparency when everything seems opaque.

Yes, a need for *the interior life*.[7]

"The interior life" includes those psychological and spiritual factors that provide us with inner strength, a sound attitude, and a sense of honesty or transparency. Different traditions encourage various approaches to strengthen or deepen the inner life.

> Our "interior," "inner," or "spiritual" life must take into account the needs and tendencies of the whole person. In addition, each of us as individuals is unique and therefore must respond in accord with his or her own uniqueness. Yet, even though this be the case, in the broad sense, there are several attitudes/ behaviors as well as individual and communal actions that are capable of nurturing the "spiritual" dimension of life.[8pp11-12]

Included among them, the ones that do have great psychological value and are therefore of interest to us here—whether we are persons of a specific faith or not—are *silence* and *solitude, friendship* and *community, humor* and *laughter* and *listening* and *reflection.*

These four essential elements of the core spiritual practices have especially sound psychological value for persons seeking to be centered in life in a way that helps them learn from the necessary stresses in life and avoid the unnecessary ones. However, the basis of the four essential elements is a recognition that, as Heschel notes, the inner life "requires education, training, reflection, contemplation. It is not enough to join others; it is necessary to build a sanctuary within, brick by brick."[9] Otherwise, we will be drawn to settle for so little in life and call this "practicality." In a similar vein, Heschel also cautions, "People are anxious to save up financial means for old age; they should also be anxious to prepare a spiritual means for old age. . . . Wisdom, maturity, tranquility do not come suddenly when we retire."[10p79]

This latter quote by Heschel surfaces periodically as we face our own challenges, darkness, stress and changes in working as medical and nursing professionals In other words, achieving wisdom, maturity and tranquility requires personal effort and asks that we be clearer on the following:

- What provides a theme and purpose for my personal life?
- What is the meaning that drives my work as a caregiver of patients or other caregivers?
- How can I continue to care for others in a professional yet deeply compassionate manner?
- How could I truly nurture my own interior life through new, creative, disciplined, and simple ways?

The steps to achieving a deeper and more resilient self requires an awareness of the four key aspects of the inner, interior, or spiritual life. And the first one, *silence and solitude*, is especially important.

Silence and Solitude

The value of silence and solitude is recognized for its purely psychological worth due to the work of psychiatrist Anthony Storr. In his work *On Solitude*, he notes the following:

Modern psychotherapists, including myself have taken as their criterion of emotional maturity the capacity of the individual to make mature relationships on equal terms. With few exceptions, psychotherapists have omitted to consider the fact that the capacity to be alone is also an aspect of emotional maturity.[11p18]

From a spiritual standpoint, long before Storr and other mental health professionals wrote positively about silence and solitude, all the major religions emphasized the value of taking out time to retreat from activity. This is clearly reflected in the writings of contemporary spiritual figures. For instance, Henri Nouwen, a spiritual writer (and incidentally also a psychologist), notes in his book *Way of the Heart* that silence and solitude are the furnace in which transformation takes place.[12p20]

In his book *The Tibetan Book of Living and Dying*, contemporary Buddhist author Sogyal Rinpoche frames such periods of silence as "meditation." He points out that slowing down the pace of our lives by ensuring we have time to stop, breathe, and see how habits and compulsions have quietly strangled us is essential. He writes:

> We are already perfectly trained . . . trained to get jealous, trained to grasp, trained to be anxious and sad and desperate and greedy, trained to react angrily to whatever provokes us. We are trained . . . to such an extent that these negative emotions rise spontaneously, without our even trying to generate them. . . . However if we devote the mind in meditation to the task of freeing itself from illusions, we will find that with time, patience, discipline, and the right training, our mind will begin to unknot itself and know the essential bliss and clarity.[13p56]

He then goes on to say the following:

> The gift of learning to meditate is the greatest gift you can give yourself in this life. For it is only through meditation that you can understand the journey to discover your true nature, and so find the stability and confidence you will need to live, and die, well. Meditation is the road to enlightenment.
>
> Our lives are lived in intense and anxious struggle, in a swirl of speed and aggression, in competing, grasping, possessing, and achieving, forever burdening ourselves with extraneous activities and preoccupations. Meditation is the exact opposite.[13p57]

Orthodox Rabbi Aryeh Kaplan expresses a similar positive sentiment regarding meditation in his book *Meditation and Kabbalah*. He acknowledges the fact that technique is similar throughout different world religions and points out that there is a lack of awareness of this tradition of meditation among practicing Jews:

> Many people [also] express surprise that the Jewish tradition contains a formal meditative system, that, at least in its outward manifestations, does resemble some of the Eastern systems. This resemblance was first noted in Zohar, which recognized the merit of the Eastern systems, but warned against their use.
>
> The fact that different systems resemble each other is only a reflection on the veracity of the technique, which is primarily one of spiritual liberation. The fact that other religions make use of it is of no more consequence than the fact that they also engage in prayer and worship. This does not make Jewish worship and prayer any less meaningful or unique, and the same is true of meditation. It is basically a technique for releasing oneself from the bonds of one's physical nature. Where one goes from there depends upon the system used.[14p3]

Whether we are Buddhist, Muslim, Jewish, Christian, Hindu, or not religious at all, though, the point is that when we speak about time in silence and solitude, or formal meditation, there is a benefit—especially for those working in the intensity of health care today.

In *The Wooden Bowl*, Clark Strand, a former Zen Buddhist monk, wrote about taking out time for meditation even though you are no longer holding onto a religious or philosophical ideology:

> All I wanted in the first place was to find the simple truth about who we are and how we ought to live. . . . I asked myself one question: Was there a way for people to slow down and experience themselves, their lives, and other people in the present moment. . . . The only thing [meditation] requires is that you be willing to remain a beginner, that you forgo achieving any expert status. . . . In other words, it requires you to maintain a spirit of lightness and friendliness regarding what you are doing. It's nothing special, but it works.[15pp2-3]

In extolling the value of being a meditative person—whether you are religious or not, does not matter in his mind—Strand goes on to say what he believes it offers all of us:

Perhaps you have had the experience of waking well-rested on a Saturday morning. Your mind is alert, but you have not yet begun to think about the day. The sun is shining in the yard and all around you is perfectly clear morning light. That alertness sustains itself without even trying. You may not even notice it except for the feeling of being rested and ready for the day.

The experience of meditation is something like that. When you meditate you are not trying to have any particular experience. You are simply awake. After having counted your breath from one to four for several minutes, quite without having aimed at that experience, you start to feel a kind of clarity and space surrounding each number as you count. It feels a little like having enough space to think, enough room to move and breathe, or simply "be."[16p96]

The benefits are certainly there if we approach such a place, not with a sense of duty, but as a time for returning to our self; it will become a gentle place of reassurance, reassessment, and peace. Time spent in silence and solitude on a regular basis can affect us in the following ways:

- Sharpen our sense of clarity about the life we are living and the choices we are making
- Enhance our attitude of simplicity
- Increase our humility and help us avoid unnecessary arrogance by allowing time to examine the defenses and games we play (these often surface for us to see during quiet times)
- Let us enjoy our relationship with ourselves more
- Decrease our dependence on the reinforcement of others
- Enable us to recognize our own anger, entitlement, greed, and cowardice
- Protect our own inner fire so that we can reach out without being pulled down
- Help us accept change and loss
- Make us more sensitive to the compulsions in our lives
- Experience the importance of love and acceptance and acknowledge the silliness and waste involved in condemning self and judging others

- Allow us to hear the gentle inner voice that reflects the spiritual sound of authenticity . . . and
- Help us to respect the need to strengthen our own inner space so that we can, in turn, be more sensitive to the . . . presence of others.

In other words, taking quiet time in solitude and silence during each day can provide us with a place to breathe deeply. . . . Yet even when we know the true value of silence and solitude, we run from it. For us, to value the quiet in our lives, we must know not only what these periods can do for us but also . . . appreciate *what price they may extract from us.* Otherwise, we will just continue to speak about silence and solitude wistfully as something wonderful and never enjoy what this well of truth and support can offer us.[16pp42–43] (Emphasis is original)

Recognizing the Challenges of Silence and Solitude

People always make time for what they want to do. When the schedule is full, they may get up early, stay up late, or set aside periods during the day—even if it turns out to limit their lunch break. So, why would we not want to set aside time for quiet periods if we feel they really have so many benefits?

A Psychological Vacuum

As well as opening us to loneliness and vulnerability, silence and solitude can form a psychological vacuum into which many feelings, memories, and impressions (which lie below the surface in the preconscious) may be encouraged to surface. At such times as these, we are being called in reflection . . . to face the truths about ourselves that for some unconscious reason we may have put aside, denied, or diminished.

Having such truths surface is not terrible, of course, especially if we remember that many of these insights will be helpful rather than harmful. The only "damage" is that which will be suffered by the false image of ourselves that we have created because we have not been willing to trust in our own inherent value. So, by spending time in silence and solitude, we will be able to see the extent to which our self-worth has, to this point, been built upon a foundation of sand. We will come to recognize that our sense of self-worth is dependent in an exaggerated way on praise by others, positive experiences we have (including ones in prayer and meditation), and a list of other past achievements. Though unpleasant, finding out this truth is still quite life-giving. Such an epiphany allows us to rediscover a sense of self and worth grounded in true self-respect. We then can come to understand that real self-respect is based on a deep, concrete trust in the inherent spiritual value of being a human person rather than on specific accomplishments or the reception of kudos from others.

Arriving at this point of insight is not a magical process. The desire to be a person who is solidly aware of self-worth no matter what others say or do, no matter what mistakes or shameful things we might do, cannot thrive just as a wishful thought. It must be welcomed and passionately sought in silence and solitude, that place in which a strong and healthy attitude toward *all* of life is formed.[16pp45–49]

Once we consider taking time to sit in silence and solitude or *zazen* in a group, we may then raise another set of objections:

The *first objection* is: "When I quiet down and try to enjoy the silence, all I do is hear the noise of my thoughts and worries. So, I know I'm not made for meditation or reflection." This is a typical objection of beginners. It needs to be handled, otherwise we will quit after a couple of minutes, no matter how many times we try.

The reality is that most of us hear noise in our minds all day long. When we sit in silence, the first important bit of information we learn is how preoccupied we are with so many things. Knowing this is helpful because it

- Helps us let the static expend itself. (Given a chance, after a while our mind calms down.)
- Gives us some indication of the type of worries we have about which we feel helpless or anxious. (We get a chance to hear what we are continually thinking.)
- Prepares us to empty our minds so we can breathe deeply, relax, and experience "the now" rather than always being caught in the past or preoccupied with the future.

So, expecting the noise and letting it move through us are two ways we can meet the objection that we are not suited or able to quietly reflect or meditate. The reality we must remember is: Many people with our personality type have found meditation wonderfully helpful. It is not just a certain type of person.

A *second objection* is: "Meditation or reflection is too hard and alien. I'm not a yogi and have found meditation or even quiet prayer uncomfortable." The response to this is simple:

- Find a quiet place (alone if possible).
- Sit up straight.
- Close your eyes or keep them slightly open looking a few feet in front of you.
- Count slow, naturally exhaled breaths from one to four and repeat the process.
- Relax and let stray thoughts move through you like a slow-moving train, repeating themes; observe objectively then let them go. . . .
- Experience living in the now.

A *third objection* comes in the form of a question: "What will this time do for me? I'm a busy person and time is too precious for me to deal with impractical exercises." There are many responses to this. For our purposes here—namely, the desire to change, grow, and be freer—the following are especially relevant:

- When we are quiet, we experience the pulls, anxieties, and conditioned responses we have going on all day but may fail to notice. So, at the very least it informs us of the nature of what blocks us from feeling at ease, flexible, open, and ready to change when necessary.
- Not only will we be able to see what absorbs us but how things we didn't realize have become our most important reference point or center of psychological/spiritual gravity.
- Once we have this information, we can take note of it and reflect on it mentally, in journaling, or with a mentor during other periods outside of the quiet time.
- Also, the peaceful times when we sit and reflect physically stops us from running, running, running, without taking

a breath, and so we experience what it means to be alive and, in the process, ask ourselves if that is where we want to focus our lives.

If it sounds like I are putting great emphasis on quiet time, I am. I have found if we give some space to ourselves and try not to judge ourselves and others harshly, and avoid panicking or trying to immediately solve a problem, but instead calm ourselves down, we will learn not to jump to quick conclusions; our usual ways of doing business (our programming) will not take hold. This will allow our habits to loosen their hold on us so we can see life—including ourselves—differently.

When people do express their gratitude for the recommendation that they take at least two minutes a day for quiet reflection first thing in the morning, they often report extending it to twenty minutes. Then they try to find another ten minutes during the day to reconnect with the experience and find another few minutes in the evening to become tranquil, give closure, and release the day before they go to sleep.

In guiding others toward using meditation as a building block to enable change, one of the other things I also notice is that it loosens people up throughout their whole day—not just during the reflection period. The more we allow our thoughts to inform, rather than frighten, depress, or anger us, the less we are grasped by our [rigid] thinking and interpretations. We are not in a vise but are instead free to use our power of observation, analysis, and curiosity to help us learn valuable lessons about life. Meditation not only frees us to be open during the period of reflection, it also produces an attitude that makes us less defensive and more intrigued with stumbles as well as triumphs. It can positively contaminate our day![17pp52–55]

Friendship and Community

As well as silence and solitude, another key aspect of the inner life is to have a well-rounded circle of friends. Psychology has long emphasized the need for humans to relate, a key element of health and happiness. For all major spiritual traditions, "community" is an essential element.

Yet, the members of that community are just as significant as the recognition that we should be part of one. As psychologist and spiritual writer Henri Nouwen recognizes: "We can take a lot of physical and even mental pain when we know that it truly makes us a part of the life we live together in the world. But when we feel cut off from the human family, we quickly lose heart."[18p33]

Research evidence has confirmed Nouwen's insights specifically concerning the relationship between "loneliness" and cardiovascular risk. Between 2004 and 2010, a group of 5397 men and women over 50 years of age were followed for new fatal and nonfatal diagnoses of heart disease and stroke. Over the 5.4 years of follow-up, 571 new cardiovascular events emerged. Findings strongly suggest that loneliness was associated with an increased risk of heart disease and stroke independent of other risk factors such as smoking and obesity. Researchers interpret findings to suggest that strategies to prevent loneliness could contribute significantly to the prevention of cardiovascular disease.[19]

For a circle of friends to be rich and to play distinctive roles at different points in our lives, we need four "types" or "voices" among them. They are the prophet, the cheerleader, the harasser, and the guide. These "voices" will increase our chances of maintaining a sense of perspective, openness, and balance. A brief description of each follows[20,21]:

The Prophet
The first of these voices which help us maintain balance and have a sense of openness is the one I shall refer to as the prophet. Contrary to what one might imagine, prophetic friends need not look or behave any differently than other types of persons who are close to us. . . . The true prophet's voice is often quiet and fleeting, but nonetheless strong. She or he is living an honest courageous life guided by truth and compassion. . . . They are trying to live out the truth, and whether knowingly or not, they follow the advice of Gandhi: "Let our first act every morning be this resolve: I shall not fear anyone on earth. I shall fear only God. I shall not bear ill-will toward anyone. I shall conquer untruth by truth and in resisting untruth, I shall put up with all suffering."

The message of prophets often involves discomfort or pain, not masochistic pain but real pain. Prophets may not directly produce conflict. Instead, like leaders in the non-violent movement, they "merely" set the stage for it, as indicated in the words of Martin Luther King, Jr.:

We who engage in nonviolent, direct action are Not the creators of tension. We merely bring to The surface the hidden tension that is already alive. We bring it out in the open, where it can be seen and dealt with. Like a boil that can never be cured so long as it is covered up but must be opened with all its ugliness to the natural medicines of air and light, injustice must be exposed, with all the tension its exposure creates, to the light of human conscience and the air of national opinion before it can be cured.

Having someone prophetic in our lives is never easy. No matter how positive we may believe the ultimate consequences will be for us, many of us still shy away from prophetic messages and would readily agree with Henry Thoreau: "If you see someone coming to do you a good deed, run for your life!" However, to seek comfort in lieu of the truth may mean that in avoiding pain, we will also avoid responding to opportunities of real value, real life. We will merely exist and eventually die without having ever really lived. . . . Prophets point! They point to the fact that it doesn't matter whether pleasure or pain is involved, the only thing that matters is . . . that we seek to see and live "the truth" because only it will set us free. In doing this, prophets challenge us to look at how we are living our lives, to ask ourselves: "To what voices am I listening when I form my attitudes and take my actions each day?"

The Cheerleader

Ironically, one of the most controversial suggestions we are making with respect to friendship is that we all need "cheerleaders." . . . Some might say that to encourage this type of friend is to run the risk of narcissism and denial. However, to balance the prophetic voices . . . we also need unabashed, enthusiastic, unconditional acceptance by certain people in our lives. Prophetic voices can and should instill appropriate guilt to break through the crusts of our denial. But guilt cannot sustain us for long. Guilt may push us to do good things because they are right, but loving encouragement will push us to do the right thing because it is natural.

The bottom line is that we cannot go it alone. We need a balance of support. We need encouragement and acceptance as much as we need the criticism and feedback that are difficult to hear. Burnout is always around the corner when we don't have people who are ready to encourage us, see our gifts clearly, and be there for us when the unrealistic demands of people and our own crazy expectations for ourselves, threaten to pull us down. Make no mistake about it, having buoyantly supportive friends may seem like a luxury, but it is rather a necessity, not to be taken lightly. The "interpersonal roads" of time are strewn with well-meaning helpers who tried to survive without such support. This is particularly true of medical and nursing professionals. Encouragement is a gift that should be treasured in today's stressful, anxious, complex world because the seeds of involvement and the seeds of burnout are the same. To be involved is to risk. And to risk without the presence of solidly supportive friends is foolhardy and dangerous.

The Harasser
When singer-activist Joan Baez was asked her opinion about Thomas Merton, she said that he was different than many of the phony gurus she had encountered in her travels. She said that although Merton took important things seriously in his life, he did not take himself too seriously. She indicated that he knew how to laugh at situations and particularly at himself [see Baez[22p45]]. On the way to taking the healthcare of others seriously, we run the danger of making an unconscious "psychological detour" by taking *ourselves* too seriously instead. The "Harasser" helps us to laugh at ourselves as a way to gain, regain and maintain perspective and conserve our energy, which is truly a gift for which to be thankful.

Spiritual Guides
The prophet, the cheerleader, and the harasser, three friends that are each part of a necessary community. The prophet enhances our sense of clarity by asking, "What voices are guiding us in life?" because many times we are unaware of the un-examined values from which we are currently operating—especially

when we are under a great deal of stress. The cheerleader generously showers us with the support we feel we need. The harasser encourages us to maintain a sense of proper perspective. Complementing these three is a cluster that, for lack of a better name, shall be referred to as "spiritual guides" . . . who listen to us carefully and don't accept the "manifest content" (what we say and do) as being equal to the "total content" (our actual intentions plus our statements and actions). Instead, they search and look for nuances in what we share with them to help us to uncover some of the "voices" that are unconsciously guiding our lives, especially the ones that make us hesitant, anxious, fearful, and willful.

To determine whether or how these voices are in our lives, several questions or statements about the composition of our circle of friends might be helpful:

- Do I have people with whom I can simply be myself?
- What type of friends do I value most? Why?
- What do I feel are the main qualities of friendship?
- List and briefly describe the friends who are now in my life.
- Describe ones who are no longer alive or present to me now but who have made an impact on my life. Why do I think they made such a difference in my life?
- Among my circle of friends, who are my personal heroes or role models?
- Who are the prophets in my life? In other words, who confronts me with the question: To what voices am I responding in life?
- Who helps me see my relationships, mission in life, and self-image more clearly? How do they accomplish this?
- Who encourages me in a genuine way through praise and a nurturing spirit?
- Who teases me into gaining a new perspective when I am too preoccupied or tied up in myself?
- When and with whom do I play different (prophetic, supportive . . .) roles as a friend? How do people receive such interactions?[1]

Having encouraging, challenging and guiding friendships in our lives, can aid in stress prevention and personal/professional growth both psychologically and spiritually.[8pp69–70]

Humor and Laughter

Like silence/solitude and friendship/community, humor and laughter are key elements in building and strengthening one's inner life. A sense of humor is a psychological trait that varies from person to person. Humor is rooted in culture, time, and place. What may be considered funny in one culture may be an insult in another or what was funny in the eighteenth century may not be funny now. Acquiring a sense of humor, *or not*, is a lifelong developmental process. Laughter, on the other hand, is the psycho-physiological expression of humor (e.g., the smile or the belly laugh). Humor and laughter can be considered as fundamentally spiritual because of their connection to joy, a spiritual state and life goal.

The mental and physical health benefits of humor and laughter have been well documented since Norman Cousins popularized the notion of laughter as medicine through his painful battle with ankylosing spondylitis.[23] Cousins checked himself into a hotel and watched Marx Brothers' movies. He discovered that 10 minutes of genuine belly laughs would give him at least two hours of pain-free sleep. Over the past three decades, research has documented the health benefits of humor and laughter. For example, the research of Miller, a cardiologist and Fry, a psychiatrist point to a possible direct link between positive emotions, particularly "mirthful laughter" and beneficial effects on the vascular system.[24] Humor was found to be a key factor correlated with longevity. Sevak et al.,[25] in a seven-year study of 66,000 adults, found sense of humor to be a key factor in reaching to age 65 and beyond.

Humor is also instrumental in connecting us to others; to friends, family, colleagues, and to those for whom we care. In contrast, medical and nursing education has advanced the notion that with respect to clinician–patient relationships, the clinician was to be a "blank slate"—reacting thoughtfully, analytically, and, most important, objectively. The power of humor in clinician–patient relationships was not traditionally studied in curricula nor encouraged in the practice arena. You may even recall the occasional instructor who cautioned against your overinvolvement with patients or against "seeming to be having too much fun" while giving care. Humor and laughter, nevertheless, are often powerful catalysts for positive change in clinical relationships.

Carla, a psychiatric nurse, had lunch duty and was assigned to dine with the same two patients, each day, John and Jill. Both patients were experiencing serious psychotic disorders and required extra supervision during mealtimes. The unit dining room had huge windows that looked onto the expressway below and the lunch table was situated near the windows. Both patients were a bit agitated at the beginning of the meal. John was most likely hearing menacing voices. Jill was eating fast and speaking rapidly and loudly. The nurse offered some distracting conversation, "Lots of traffic on the expressway!" Jill stood, pointed to the traffic and exclaimed, "John, John, see that truck down there—it is a van and I own it, I own a van company, John. See it, see it!" John continued eating and finally stared directly at Jill, "Get your van off my expressway!" he directed. The nurse spontaneously laughed out loud, then so did both the patients. What followed was a rather rational conversation as if the three were merely dining companions. This incident had long term benefits. It created a closer bond between the nurse and patients and enabled the nurse to reach and comfort the patients more effectively when their symptoms were worsening. It also gave the nurse a broader perspective about the power of humor and connection in the work of caring.

The unusually high level of stress experienced by medical and nursing professionals in the recent pandemic signals that we need to do more to help professionals build resilience. Spike and Carlin[26] recommend that medical practitioners cultivate a "humorous outlook on life." They cite Sigmund Freud's belief that humor conserves psychic energy. They conclude that "the way in which affect can influence how one sees and event, coloring it so as to seem either funny or sad, is one of the most important determinants of resilience."[26p286]

In his book, *Between Heaven and Mirth,* James Martin[27] points to the following benefits of humor in developing not only deeper relationships with others but also with oneself. He asserts that.

- Humor is a tool to attract people; it has an evangelizing quality.
- Humor promotes humility, resulting in not taking ourselves so seriously.
- Humor speaks truth; it shocks us into dealing with reality; it lays bare the point.
- Humor enables courage and the speaking of truth to power.
- Humor deepens relationships with the self, others. and God.

- Humor is welcoming; it is hospitable.
- Humor can heal both body and mind and promote relaxation.
- Humor opens our minds to other possibilities.
- Humor is fun and everyone needs some fun in their lives.

Each of these characteristics of humor can enhance moments of solitude and build friendship and community in our efforts to strengthen our inner life.

During our moments of solitude and silence, it may be well to recall Thomas More's Prayer for Good Humor,[28] written while he was imprisoned in the Tower of London waiting to be executed. It is a useful tool for daily reflection as we consider the fourth key aspect of the inner, spiritual life—listening and reflection.

Prayer for Good Humor
by St. Thomas More

Grant me, O Lord, good digestion, and also something to digest.

Grant me a healthy body, and the necessary good humor to maintain it.

Grant me a simple soul that knows to treasure all that is good and that doesn't frighten easily as the sight of evil, but rather finds the means to put things back in their place.

Give me a soul that knows not boredom, grumblings, sighs and laments, nor excess of stress because of that obstructing thing called "I."

Grant me, O Lord, a good sense of humor.

Allow me the grace to be able to take a joke, to discover in life a bit of joy, and to be able to share it with others.

Listening and Reflection

Being as open as we can in both meditation and in our relationships can teach us a great deal about ourselves if we really *listen* "(a very important word). In the effort to be a true listener to whatever provides greater awareness and inner strength is not something to be taken lightly. Becoming a listening-reflective person does take some sense of structured intention rather than just motivation and good will. It involves

1. Finding time to reflect.
2. Selecting meaningful events in our day and life to reflect upon.
3. Reliving those events in our minds.
4. Learning what we can from these events, given our desires, goals, and philosophy of life.
5. Enlivening the learning through action.

An elaboration of the five-step process follows.

> *Time*: A little time is needed to reflect on one's day. If we rush through life, without thought we will know it. One alarming sign is when we ask: "Where did the time go?" When our life is passing like a blur, it does not mean that we live very *active* lives. What it does show is that we are leading *busy* lives. The difference between "active" and "busy" is that the former includes reflection and is directed, whereas the later feels out of control and does not seem purposeful or meaningful.
>
> *Select*: To make reflection useful and not just a time to preoccupy ourselves, to worry, or to let our mind wander, we should choose *specific* events or interactions during the day that caused a significant reaction.
>
> *Enter*: We should then revisit the events so we can relive them. This time as we experience the event, we can observe our reactions, note them, and see what themes or understanding we can glean. (Remember, do not *blame* others, or *condemn* self, just neutrally observe and seek to analyze.)
>
> *Learn*: Given what we understand and what our core beliefs (psychological or spiritual) are about life, what did we learn from this reflection? Often when we have values, we can see how we followed those values or ignored them.
>
> *Action*: Finally, learning is only important when it changes the way we live. How we act on our new learning is crucial. And it cannot be action that is immature such as, when you feel a person has let you down, making the vow, *I'll never trust him again!* Instead, using the example just cited, you must consider what about the interaction led you to be naïve and to put more trust in a certain person than he

or she could bear. So, in other words, action must be based on insight that we have about our *own* behavior, beliefs, and thoughts. Otherwise, the results will be just a sophisticated form of pouting, projecting, and avoidance of self-understanding.[17pp57–58] (Emphasis in original)

When we become true listeners, we recognize that there are many voices calling us of which we are not aware. The sources of them may be good in their own way and include the desire to succeed, be well off financially, be admired, be spectacularly effective, or be loved. The sources can be career, family upbringing, society, the health care system, politics, or culture. When we make daily decisions that affect us in the long run, knowing which sources are primary can help us to decide the best course of action in any given situation. And so, one of the positive outcomes of a strong inner life is achieving a high level of self-awareness.

Naturally, there are many other elements and "fruits" of a strong inner life. As has been noted, having a strong community of friends and knowing the benefit of taking out time in silence and solitude and having a healthy sense of humor certainly are among them. Reserving time to further explore your history and current sense of the role of religion and/or spirituality in your life, regardless of whether you are presently a person of faith, can also be helpful.[29,30]

A guide to clarifying your spiritual life map is provided in Box 4.1.

No matter how you begin to sensitize yourself to this area, the information can provide additional self-knowledge and set the stage for the development of a richer self-care protocol and a more fulfilling professional life. As otherwise noted,

> the state of our interior life *does* make a difference to others. When we have a gentle, healthy, and strong inner life, we are part of the healing stillness in the world which offers places of hope to all who suffer and yearn for justice, solace, and encouragement. But if we, like so many others, do not feel at home within ourselves, and by ourselves, we will then add to the sense in the world that nowhere is there a safe and good place.[8pp14–16]

Box 4.1 Clarifying Your Spiritual Life Map

1. Do you consider yourself a spiritual person? If so, explain.
2. What role did spirituality and/or religion play in your family growing up? What role does it play now?
3. When the word *God* is used, what images come to mind?
4. When you are under stress, depressed, anxious, lost, angry, joyful, happy, elated, or experiencing other strong emotions, does God or spirituality play a role for you when these states are present?
5. If you are part of an organized religion, how does this affect the way you function as a physician, nurse, or allied health professional? How does it affect your personal life?
6. If you have a personal relationship with God, how does this affect the way you live your life?
7. What type of spiritual practices do you have, and has their meaningfulness and/or form changed in recent years?
8. Do you seek to read the sacred scripture of one or more of the major world religions or spiritual books? What do you seek to get out of them? How has this reading list changed over the years?
9. Given your own beliefs, how do you interact with others of different beliefs? Do you find their literature, practices, or beliefs a help to you in any way?
10. When you are under stress, what parts of your spirituality— if any—provide you with a sense of relief and perspective?

References

1. Koenig HG. *Religion, Spirituality and Health: The Research and Clinical Implications*. Bern, German: International Scholarly Research Network Psychiatry; 2012.
2. Pargament K. Religious methods of coping: resources for conservation and transformation of significance. In: Shafranske EP, ed. *Religion and the Clinical Practice of Psychology*. Washington, DC: American Psychiatric Association; 1996: 28–49.

3. Hood R, Spilka B, Budsberger B, Gorsuch R. *The Psychology of Religion.* New York, NY: Guilford Press; 1986.

4. Benson H. *Timeless Healing: The Power and Biology of Beliefs.* New York, NY: Scribner; 1996.

5. Emory N. Tracking the mind–body connection: an interview with Herbert Benson. *Brain World.* https://brainworldmagazine.com/tracking-mind-body-connection-interview-dr-herbert-benson/https://www.guideposts.org/inspiration/miracles/gods-grace/father-james-martin-on-the-sacredness-of-laughter. Published November 7, 2019. Accessed June 2, 2020.

6. Johnston-Taylor E. *Fast Facts About Religion for Nurses: Implications for Patient Care.* New York, NY: Springer; 2019.

7. Dubois D. Renewal of prayer. *Lumen Vitae.* 1983;38(3):273–274.

8. Wicks R. *After 50.* Mahwah, NJ: Paulist Press; 1997.

9. Heschel AJ. "On Prayer," *Conservative Judaism.* 1970;25:1.

10. Heschel AJ. *The Insecurity of Freedom.* New York, NY: Farrar, Straus, and Giroux; 1951.

11. Storr A. *On Solitude.* New York, NY: Bantam, 1988.

12. Nouwen H. *The Way of the Heart.* New York, NY: Seabury/Harper Collins; 1981. 20.

13. Rinpoche S. *The Tibetan Book of Living and Dying.* New York, NY: Harper Collins; 2002.

14. Kaplan A. *Meditation and Kabbalah.* York Beach, ME: Samuel Weiser; 1982.

15. Strand C. *The Wooden Bowl.* New York, NY: Hyperion; 1998.

16. Wicks R. *Living Gentle, Passionate Life.* Mahwah, NJ: Paulist Press; 1998.

17. Wicks R. *Simple Changes.* Allen, TX: Thomas More; 2000.

18. Nouwen H. *Making All Things New.* New York: Harper and Row; 1981.

19. Valtorta NK, Kanaan M, Gilbody S, Hanratty B. Loneliness, social isolation and risk of cardiovascular disease in the English longitudinal study of ageing. *European Journal of Preventive Cardiology.* 2018;25(13):1389–1396.

20. Wicks R, Hamma R. *Circle of Friends.* Notre Dame, IN: AMP; 1996.

21. Wicks R. *Touching the Holy: Ordinariness, Self-Esteem and Friendship.* Notre Dame, IN: AMP; 1992.

22. Baez J. Merton the prophet. In: Wilkes P, ed. *Merton: By Those Who Knew Him Best* San Francisco, CA: Harper; 1984: 41–46.

23. Cousins N. *Anatomy of an Illness as Perceived by the Patient.* New York, NY: W. W. Norton; 1979.

24. Miller M, Fry WF. The effect of mirthful laughter on the human cardiovascular system. *Medical Hypotheses.* 2009;73(5):636.

25. Sevak S, Romundstad S, Homan J. A 7-year prospective study of sense of humor and mortality in an adult county population. *International Journal of Psychiatry in Medicine.* 2010;40(2):125–146.

26. Spike J, Carlin N. Ethical decisions: stress and distress in medicine. In: Figley C, Huggard P, Rees CE, eds. *First Do No Harm: Understanding and Promoting Physician Stress Resilience.* New York, NY: Oxford University Press; 2013: 281–293.

27. Martin J. *Between Heaven and Mirth: When Joy, Humor and Laughter Are at the Heart of Spiritual Life.* New York, NY: Harper Collins; 2011.

28. Hallett PE. The English Prayers of St. Thomas More *Written when He Was a Prisoner in the Tower of London in 1534.* West Conshohocken, PA: Templeton Publishers; 1995.

29. Ciarrocchi J. *Counseling Problem Gamblers: Self-Regulation Manual for Individual and Family Therapy.* San Diego, CA: Academic Press; 2002.

30. Wicks R. *Seeds of Sensitivity: Deepening Your Spiritual Life.* Notre Dame, IN: AMP, 1995.

FIVE

The Simple Care of a Hopeful Heart

Developing a Personally Designed Self-Care Protocol

Objectives

- Assess workaholism, happiness and satisfaction in career and life.
- Explore basic stress management strategies for overall health.
- Respect self and others as foundational to managing secondary stress.
- Differentiate toxic work environments from intense work environments.
- Design a personally tailored self-care protocol.

I wanted to change the world. But I have found that the only thing one can be sure of changing is oneself.

—Aldous Huxley

After experiencing 2 years of extreme job stress in a failing healthcare organization compulsively working long hours and dealing with significant family issues, Marta took a "self-care plunge." She made an appointment to see a therapist. "What am I doing here?" she silently wondered as she sat in the therapist's waiting area. "I just need to pull myself together and move on." Just as Marta was about to abandon the appointment, the door opened, and Dr. Paul welcomed her into his office. Marta sat on the couch across from Dr. Paul who opened the conversation, "Tell me what brought you here." Marta's mind raced to find a reply, instead she began to cry, then sob. She tried to speak, to gather her thoughts but the flood of tears washed every rational thought away. She cried for at least half an hour and was thinking to herself how wasteful this was. Afterall, these sessions were expensive, and all this crying was wasting time—a typical response from Marta who was driven to succeed—cost effectively. Dr. Paul just sat supportively, saying nothing, handing Marta a tissue from time to time. When the crying ended, Marta tried to answer Dr. Paul's initial question. She described her extreme work and family issues and admitted needing "guidance." She could not bring herself to say the word help. Dr. Paul listened intently and then said, "This is a good beginning. I will see you next week—same time?" And the weekly sessions continued for the next five years as Marta learned to adjust her perspective and take better care of herself.

Health care is one of the few professions where it is socially acceptable to ignore your family, your nonwork life, *yourself.* Workaholism and burnout are increasingly serious problems among physicians, physician assistants (PA), and nurses. For physicians it begins during residency. Shaufeli et al.[1] studied workaholism and related variables among 2,115 medical residents. Using standard assessment scales, they determined that "working excessively" combined with "working compulsively" results in workaholism and its attendant negative results. Compared to their "hard-working" colleagues, workaholic medical residents

- Exhibited higher levels of exhaustion and recovered less well,
- Showed a strong tendency to relate to patients in a more callous or cynical manner,
- Believed that they accomplished less than their counterparts, and
- By their own assessment, performed poorly delivering medical care.

As a prelude to these recent findings, Gabbard and Menninger theorized many years ago with respect to physicians as to why there might be a predisposition to workaholism and burnout:

> The demands of practice are a convenient rationalization. Physicians work long hours to deny dependency, to eradicate any trace of aggression or destructiveness that they fear others may suspect; win the unconditional love and approval of colleagues, patients, and community; to maintain complete control; and to conquer the terror of death.[2p35]

Whether their theory is correct or not, care must be taken not to be driven in one's career to the extent that everything else loses value and accordingly does not receive the attention it should.

In an extensive review of studies focusing on the work life PAs by Essary et al., the existing data reveals

- Burnout among PAs is higher in specialties such as primary care, hospice and palliative care, oncology, and primary care.
- Despite reports of burnout in specific specialties, job and career satisfaction remain high.

The authors speculate that the adaptable nature of the PA role "lends itself to specialty transition which may serve as a buffer against the long-term effects of burnout."[3] They also indicate that much more research is needed on the tenor of PA work-life experiences.

In a study of 1,781 nurses, Andreassen et al.[4] investigated the relationship between workaholism and negative work-related incidents including self-harm incidents like dozing at work or while driving, harming patients, or mishaps with equipment. They found that workaholism was the most consistent predictor of

- Working despite being ill thus increasing the inevitability of negative work events.
- Impaired mental health and accident proneness.
- Diminished recovery after long hours of work.
- Obsessiveness, which contributes to increased self-reporting of negative work-related incidents.

Andreassen et al. concluded that "workaholism is consistently and positively associated with negative work-related incidents, even after controlling for various demographic and work-related variables, and sleep duration."[4p379]

Although being a healing professional is a wonderful life commitment, unless care is taken to ensure that the rest of one's life is fulfilling as well, one's life becomes too narrow, limited, and eventually distorted. This can have a negative impact not only on oneself but also on family life and other interpersonal relations.

With respect to the COVID-19 pandemic, burnout and secondary stress among clinicians is now considered a parallel pandemic. Dzau et al.,[5] of the National Academy of Medicine, Action Collaborative on Clinician Well-Being and Resilience, recommend that every health care organization have a chief wellness officer with a voice at the highest level of the organization. There should be wellness programs for staff and clinicians should be encouraged to speak out about their work conditions and risks. Health care organizations should also be supporting the self-care efforts of the clinical staff. Finally, the authors recommend a post–COVID-19 national epidemiological tracking program to measure clinician well-being.[5] Investing in clinician well-being will go a long way to improve not only the quality of care but also the long-term health and viability of health care organizations.

In addition to workaholism and the narrowing of one's horizon so that outside interests, family, and even self are left out, there is the added problem of denial. Most health care professionals would deal with the dangers of burnout or vicarious posttraumatic stress disorder if they were aware of them. They would also view the elements of stress management in a more respectful and serious manner. Stress management includes basic elements (Box 5.1) of which we are aware at some level but do not really "know" at the level of true commitment. When this is so, people who are in intense helping roles pay for this in terms of psychological and physical health—not to mention the havoc it wreaks in the family and on one's necessary social outlets. If people do not pay for ignoring stress immediately, they do so eventually. The problem with "eventually" is that as in many psychophysical disorders in which psychological stress produces physical changes over time, the damage done that seems so benign or reversible initially becomes, after a period of time, more or less permanent. At that point, even when stress is reduced and personal is self-care enriched, the physical harm already incurred will have chronic implications for the rest of one's life.

Another reality that we must deal with is that

> the self is limited. It has only so much energy. If it is not renewed, then depletion will take place. Too often we do not avail ourselves of the type of activities that truly renew us. When this occurs we run a greater risk that we will unnecessarily lose perspective and burn out, which is not only sad for us but for the people we are in a position to help in our circle of family, friends, and coworkers.[6p46]

Sometimes, however, a rude awakening is required for us to realize how far we have drifted from a balanced life.

Box 5.1 The Basics of Stress Management

Physical Health

1. Sleep: Without enough sleep the quality of what you do will decrease; rising early requires going to bed at a reasonable hour.

2. Food: Eating three light meals, at a reasonable pace, and being mindful of the nutritional value of what you eat is one of the best ways to keep weight down and nourishment and energy up.

3. Exercise: Taking a fairly brisk walk each day is a good minimum exercise. Doing it on a consistent basis is better than some irregular or future extensive exercise plan which we fail at and feel guilty about.

4. Leisure: Relaxing with your feet up and/or being involved in activities that provide genuine enjoyment are not niceties of physical health. Rather, they are undervalued but essential building blocks to good health. Leisure helps us "flow" with life's joys and problems in a more accepting philosophical way.

5. Pacing: Taking a little more time to get to a place makes the trip more relaxing; stopping every hour or hour and a half to get out of the car and stretch on long trips makes the trip a lot more enjoyable and helps increase stamina. Likewise, taking breaks when you feel the need makes your productivity better. The important lesson here is to use any technique necessary to slow yourself down so you don't rush to the grave missing the scenery in your life along the way.

Psychological Stability

1. Laughter: If laughter is good medicine, then surely laughing at yourself is healing. We all tend to take ourselves too seriously. So, doing something about this can significantly reduce unnecessary stress and help improve one's perspective on self and life.

2. Values: Know what is important and what isn't; by knowing what you believe to be really important you can choose easily and well between alternatives.

3. Control: Be careful to discern between what you can control and what you can't; while worrying about something when it happens is natural, continuing to preoccupy yourself with it is not. When you catch yourself worrying endlessly, tease yourself that you must be "the world's best worrier." Then plan what you can do about it, and let it go. If and when it comes up again; review the process until it lessens or stops. This technique may need a good deal of practice for it to "take root" in your attitude.

4. Self-Appreciation: Reflect on what gifts . . . [have been] given you, recall them each day in detail (make a list if you have to on paper), and be grateful for them by promising to nurture and share them—not in a compulsive manner but in a generous way. By this I mean have low expectations that people will respond as you would wish or appreciate your efforts. However, simultaneously still try to maintain high hopes that you can appreciate . . . multiple measures of "success" in your work so you don't miss the good that is occurring before you because of a narrow success-oriented viewpoint. For instance, too often we measure what we achieve at the end of a process and fail to see or value appropriately all of the good we did along the way.

5. Involvement . . . Not Over-Involvement: Be active in what you feel is meaningful (the kind of things you would be pleased to reflect on at the very end of life—not necessarily those things that others might feel are impressive or important). Assertiveness on your part both to volunteer to be involved in what you believe is good and to say no to demands that aren't, is also an essential part of increasing your involvement in stimulating activities and curbing (wherever possible) ones that are personally draining.

6. Support Group: Have people in your life who care; contact them frequently by phone and in writing as well as in person. Ideally, among this group should be a variety of psychologically healthy friends who can challenge, support, encourage, teach, and make you laugh.

7. Escape: There are times when we should "run away" because facing things directly in all of our relationships all the time would be debilitating. To do this you can use novels, breaks during the day, movies, walks, hobbies (fishing, bicycle riding, etc.).

8. Be Spontaneous: A small creative action or change during the day or week can make life much more fun. This is a lot more practical than waiting for a yearly vacation.

9. Be Careful of Negativity: Often we hear negative comments like thunder and praise like a whisper. Use self-talk to catch your own negative tendencies (i.e., to see things in black-and-white terms, to exaggerate the negative, to let one negative event contaminate the whole day or week, or to discount other positive events). Then answer these thoughts with more accurate positive ones. For example, if you feel slightly depressed and check your thinking, you may see that because one thing went wrong today, you are saying to yourself that you are really a failure at what you do. By recognizing this exaggeration as nonsense, you can tell yourself more correctly that you made a mistake, not that you are a mistake! Following this, you can then recall successes you have had and bring to mind the faces of those who have been grateful for your presence in their lives. This will show you the face of [love] . . . in the world and help break the back of the strong seamless negative thinking you are under at the time. Remember, negative thinking takes a good deal of energy. Stop it, and a great deal of energy will be freed up for growth and enjoyment.

10. Check Your Individual Balance in the Areas of:
   a. stimulation and quiet,
   b. reflection and action,
   c. work and leisure,

> d. self-care and care of others,
> e. self-improvement and patience,
> f. future aspirations and present positive realities,
> g. involvement and detachment.
>
> Source: Wicks RJ, *Touching the Holy: Ordinariness, Self-Esteem and Friendship.* Notre Dame, IN: AMP; 1992. Used with permission.

Wicks vouches for this personally:

Several years ago, a very close friend of mine in his early forties was dying, from brain cancer. He was outrageous and we constantly teased one another. Even though he was dying, this did not stop.

He had been living in New York and I hadn't seen much of him in the years since I was the best man at his wedding. When he was hospitalized in Philadelphia to undergo experimental treatment, I visited him. When I came to visit, he had already been there for almost two weeks.

When I inquired about his health, he shared a summary of his condition, which included loss of short-term memory. So, I said to him: "You mean you can't remember what happened yesterday?" He said: "No."

Then I smiled and said: "So, you don't remember me coming in and sitting here with you each day for five hours for the past two weeks?" He looked at me, hesitated for a second or two, grinned widely, and said . . . well I can't share exactly what he said . . . but we both had a good laugh over it.

One of the things he did surprise me with, though, was a question that really helped me put my activities in perspective. He asked: "What good things are you doing now?" As I started to launch into an obsessive (naturally well-organized) list of my recent academic and professional accomplishments, he interrupted me by saying: "No, not that stuff. I mean what really good things have you done? When have you gone fishing last? What museums have you visited lately? What good movies have you seen in the past month?" The "good things" he was speaking about the last time I saw him alive were different from the ones I, in my arrogant good health, thought about. Unfortunately, I have a lot of company in this regard.[6p50]

A self-care protocol varies from person to person and differs according to one's stage of life. As Baker notes,

> there are many ways to practice self-care. No one model exists in terms of definition, meaning, significance, or application. Differences between individuals relate to personal history, gender, and personality, and within-individual differences relate to developmental stage, or changing needs. Such differences influence the substance and process of self-care. For one person at a particular stage of life, self-care might involve maintaining a very active schedule and hiring a housekeeper. For another person, or for the same person at a different stage, self-care might involve considerable amounts of quiet, uncommitted personal time and tending one's own home.[7pp18-19]

Because a self-care protocol needs to be tailored to the individual, it is helpful to have a large pool of possibilities from which to choose. The list that follows is designed to spur thinking around what could comprise a self-care protocol in your own case. Knowing which elements you might entertain as part of a self-care protocol and questions to ponder in the overall development of it are both good initial steps in engendering self-respect, rejecting the compulsive rat race of professional life and taking responsibility for yourself.

Elements of a Self-Care Protocol

Taking the time to focus on the following basic elements of self-care necessitates that we step back from our work routine to regain perspective and engage in ongoing self-renewal. As you peruse the list, think about if and when you chose to engage in any of these elements:

- Quiet walks by yourself
- Time and space for meditation
- Spiritual and recreational reading—including the diaries and biographies of those you admire
- Light exercise . . .
- Opportunities to laugh offered by movies, cheerful friends, etc.

- A hobby such as gardening, painting, or needlework
- Telephone calls to family and friends who inspire and tease you
- Involvement in projects that renew
- Listening to music you enjoy[1p80]

Other simple steps at self-care and renewal might include the following:

- Visiting a park or hiking
- Having family or friends over for dinner or evening coffee
- Going to the library or a mega-bookstore to wander the stacks and visit the coffee bar
- Shopping for little, inexpensive things that would be fun to have
- Taking a leisurely bath rather than a quick shower
- Daydreaming
- Watching a funny movie or going to a comedy club
- Forming a "dining club" in which you have lunch once a month with a friend or sibling
- Sending e-mail to friends especially, to reconnect
- Listening to a mystery book on tape
- Reading poetry out loud
- Staying in bed later than usual on a day off
- Having a leisurely discussion with your spouse or partner over morning coffee
- Watching an old movie
- Making love with your spouse or partner
- Reading a magazine, you have never read before
- Fixing a small garden with bright cheery flowers
- Telephoning someone with whom you have not spoken in ages
- Playing the music of a singer or musician you love
- Taking a short walk (without the earphones) before and after work and/or during lunchtime
- Visiting a diner and having a cup of tea and a piece of pie
- Going on a weekend retreat at a local spirituality center so you can walk, reflect, eat when you want, read if you like, and just renew yourself
- Arranging to spend a couple of days by yourself in your own home without family or friends just to be alone without a schedule or the needs or agendas of others
- Getting a copybook, and each day writing some of your random thoughts and impressions

- Asking yourself: What brings you to life? What enlivens your spirit? [8pp80–81]

Professionals also have the opportunity for continuing education, research and writing, collaboration with colleagues, mentoring—both receiving and offering it, going on a professional or spiritual mini-retreat, and so on; the list is endless.

Think about your daily schedule including days that you are not scheduled to work. Make a brief list of how your full day goes, including the number of work hours, time at home in the evening or on weekends, and how many hours you sleep. Now, consider the self-care elements list and think about where you can intentionally and/or spontaneously put some of these elements into your schedule on a regular basis. Despite how you have operated in the past, only you have the control and power to restructure your time to include self-care, each day, week, month, and year.

Questions to Ponder in the Development of a Self-Care Protocol

Time is a precious commodity for health care professionals. How we allot it, prioritize it, and with whom we share it all say a great deal about us and the way we live our lives as you may have noticed as you reviewed the self-care elements. In the words of the Dalai Lama from his book *The Path to Tranquility*, "It is very wrong for people to feel deeply sad when they lose some money, yet when they waste the precious moments of their lives they do not have the slightest feeling of repentance."[9p73] Yet, for a physician, nurse, or PA, wasting time implies a violation. The feeling may be, if I take out time for myself, for leisure, it may not be "time well spent." Instead, this leisure could be viewed as wrong given all the demands of sick people or, at the very least, this leisure must be earned by having spent a long rotation without any real break. To counter this kind of thinking, one must first explore the options available to develop a self-care protocol that is a necessary source of constant renewal, so that care for others can be done in a quality fashion.

Once the self-care elements are reviewed, how they are used is crucial. This is the challenge: *How do we formulate a self-care protocol that we are likely to use beneficially and regularly rather than in spurts?* To ensure that an ongoing systematic program is in place, it is necessary to ask yourself several questions first. This is to avoid the dangers, on the one hand, of being unrealistic in developing a protocol and, on the other, of not being creative and expansive enough. Responding to such questions will set the stage for designing a personal self-care protocol based on the questionnaire that appears in Box 5.2. The following are questions to ponder as you move toward developing at least a beginning self-care protocol:

- Given changes in the health care system that may have resulted in more patient hours, lower status, greater chance for litigation, generally lower financial reward given the importance of the work, and overall insecurity at many levels, what creative ways have you developed to ensure that you do not lose sight of the wonders of health *care* and the important role you play in it?
- When someone says "self-care," what image comes to mind? What are the positive and negative aspects of this image? In terms of importance and how realistic it is to develop your own self-care protocol, where do you stand?
- What do you believe medical and nursing professionals need to do in terms of self-care that is different or beyond other types of caregivers?
- How do you balance the time spent alone for personal renewal with time interacting with key members of your interpersonal network (prophet, cheerleader, harasser, and inspirational friend) who are also necessary to help you keep a healthy perspective?
- Self-care and self-knowledge go hand in hand. What types of activities (i.e., structured reflection at the end of a day, informal debriefing of oneself during the drive home, journaling, mentoring, therapy, spiritual guidance, reading, etc.) in which you are involved will help you develop a systematic and ongoing analysis of how you are progressing in life?
- What types of exercise (running, walking, the gym, swimming, etc.) do you enjoy, and believe would be realistic for you on a regular basis?
- Who is in your circle of friends to provide you with encouragement, challenge, perspective, laughter, and inspiration? What ways do you ensure that you have contact with them?

Box 5.2 Self-Care Protocol Questionnaire

Please note: This material is for your own use. There is a tendency on the part of some to be quick, terse, and often global in their responses. Such defensiveness, although natural, limits the helpfulness of completing this questionnaire to gain as full an awareness as possible of your current profile and the personal goals you plan to develop for a realistic yet appropriately balanced and rich self-care program. Consequently, in preparing this personally designed protocol, the more clear, specific, complete, imaginative, and realistic your responses are to the questions provided, the more useful the material will be in integrating it into your schedule.

1. List healthy nutritional practices that you currently have in place.

2. What are specific realistic ways to improve your eating/drinking (of alcoholic beverages) habits?

3. What physical exercise do you presently get, and when is it scheduled during the week?

4. What changes do you wish to make in your schedule in terms of time, frequency, and variety with respect to exercise?

5. Where are the periods for reflection, quiet time, meditation, mini-breaks alone, opportunities to center yourself, and personal debriefing times now in your schedule?

6. Given your personality style, family life, and work situation, what changes would you like to make in your schedule to make it more intentional and balanced with respect to processing what comes to the fore in your time spent alone or in silence?

7. How much, what type, and how deeply and broadly do you read at this point?

8. What would you like to do to increase variety or depth in your reading, research, and continuing education pursuits?

9. List the activities present in your nonworking schedule not previously noted here. Along with the frequency/time, list changes to this schedule that you believe would further

enrich you personally/professionally as well as have a positive impact, in turn, on your family, colleagues, and overall social network.

Activities Frequency/Time Now Allotted or Planned to Change/Improvement
Leisure time with:
Spouse/Significant Other
Children
Parents
Family members
Friends
Going to movies
Watching TV
Visiting museums
 Sports
Attending concerts/plays
Listening to music
Hiking, biking, walking, or swimming
Making telephone calls to family and friends Hobbies (gardening, coin collecting, etc.)
Eating out for dinner, Shopping
Going to libraries, bookstores, coffee shops Sending e-mail to friends
Making love
Journaling
Continuing education
Vacations
Spending long weekends away
Meditation/reflection/sitting zazen
Religious rituals
Leisurely baths
Massage
Other activities not listed above:

_____

_____

_____

_____

10. What are the ways you process strong emotions (i.e., anger, anxiety, deep sadness, confusion, fear, emotional "highs" or the desire to violate boundaries for reasons of personal/ sexual/financial/power gratifications)?

11. Where in your schedule do you regularly undertake such emotional processing?

12. What would you like to do to change the extent and approaches you are now using for self-analysis/debriefing of self?

13. Who comprise the interpersonal anchors in your life?

14. What do you feel is lacking in your network of friends?

15. What are some reasonable initiatives you wish to undertake to have a richer network?

16. What are your sleep/rest habits now?

17. If you are not getting enough sleep/rest, what are some realistic ways to ensure you get more?

Note: This is just a partial questionnaire. Please feel free to include, analyze, and develop a plan for improvement and integration of other aspects of self-care. Also, review your answers at different points to see what resistances to change come up and how you can face them in new creative ways by yourself or with the help of a friend, colleague, mentor, or professional counselor or therapist.

- The balance between work and leisure, professional time, and personal time, varies from person to person. What is the ideal balance for you? What steps have you taken to ensure this balance is kept? What do you do when the balance is disrupted?
- There is a Russian proverb that says: "When you live next to the cemetery, you can't cry for everyone who dies." Self-care involves not getting pulled into the dramatic emotions, fears, and anger that pervade health care settings. What are the self-care elements that support a healthy sense of detachment?
- Being too conservative or being a procrastinator versus being impulsive or too quick to act in the clinical setting are extremes that can be dangerous. How do you maintain a sense of balance that prevents your compulsive involvement in either of these extremes?

- How do you prepare for change, which is such a natural part of the health care setting and clinical work?
- What is the best way to balance stimulation and time in silence and solitude, so you do not have constant stimulation on the one hand or isolation and preoccupation with self on the other?
- How do you process "unfinished business" (past events, hurts, fears, failures, lost relationships, etc.) in your life so you have enough energy to deal with the challenges and the joys in front of you?
- What or whom do you number among the stable forces in your life that are anchors for your own sense of well-being and self-care?
- In what way do you ensure that your goals are challenging and high but not unrealistic and deflating?
- What self-care steps do you have to take because of your gender or race that others of a different race or gender do not have to do?
- How has your experience set habits in motion that make self-care a challenge in some ways?
- What self-care steps are more important at this stage of your life than they were at earlier life stages?
- What emotional and physical "red flags" are you experiencing that indicate you must take certain self-care steps so as not to burn out, violate boundaries, medicate yourself in unhealthy ways, withdraw when you should not, verbally attack patients or colleagues, or drown yourself in work?
- What do you *already* do in terms of self-care? In each of the following areas, what have you found to be most beneficial: physically, socially, professionally, financially, psychologically, and spiritually?
- Are your holidays and vacations appropriately spaced and sufficient for your needs? What is the most renewing way for you to spend this time?
- Are you also conscious of the need for "daily holidays" involving a brief tea or coffee break, a short walk, playing with the children in the evening, or visiting one's friends or parents?
- What is the next step you need to take in developing your self-care protocol? How do you plan to bring this about?

Responding to these questions can improve self-knowledge in ways that aid in burnout prevention. Your responses will also increase sensitivity to how you live your life in a way that enables you to flourish personally and become more faithful and passionate professionally. Once again, the way one moves through the day depends a great deal on personality style. *Burnout is not a function of the amount of work but rather how we perceive work and interact with people as we do it.* As previously noted, burnout is a sequela to working excessively and compulsively at the same time. For example, some people complain that they are so busy that they do not have time to breathe. Others, with the same intense schedule and workload express how happy they are that they are involved in so many challenging projects.

Some of us love exercise and thrive on it. Others are more sedentary in their existence. All of us, though, want to be physically healthy. Not everyone enjoys outdoor activities and vacations packed with touring new sites and experiencing adventures in different parts of the country or world. Some of us prefer the back yard, a leisurely walk, an artist's easel, a fishing pole, or a good book and a familiar restaurant. However, all of us need to have time away at different points.

The differences among us are many. That is why each self-care protocol should be uniquely personal in its development to be both realistic and effective. Most importantly is that we have a self-care protocol in place to use as a guide every day. There can be no rationalizations nor excuses for not doing this. Not to have a personal self-care protocol is not only courting disaster in our personal and professional lives; it is also, at its core, an act of profound disrespect for yourself. One of the greatest gifts we can share with our coworkers and patients is a sense of our own peace and self-respect. However, you cannot share what you do not have.

Finally, when we speak about self-care and self-nurturing, we are not referring to another intense program that just adds more stress to life in the name of reducing it. We are instead referring to a protocol that addresses the needs of not only mind and emotions but also body and spirit. With respect to nurturing the body, Domar and Dreher emphasize the following.

> True body-nurture absolutely includes physical activity and sound nutrition but not compulsive exercise and onerous dietary restriction. True body-nurture is also much more than exercise and nutrition. It includes the following actions and ideas:

- Deep diaphragmatic breathing
- A regular practice of relaxation
- Cognitive restructuring of body-punishing thoughts into thoughts of compassion and forgiveness
- Delight in the sensual and sexual pleasures of the body
- A sane, balanced, non-shame-based relationship with food
- Health-promoting behaviors, such as stopping smoking, use of alcohol only in moderation, and regular visits to the physician for preventive care
- A profound regard for the sacredness of the body, including all its functions, imperfections, idiosyncrasies, and wonders.[10p98]

This overall approach to body nurture combined with mind and spirit approaches, addressed thus far, will help in developing an attitude and behaviors that will improve health and increase personal and professional well-being. Completing the Self-Care Protocol Questionnaire in Box 5.2 will assist in focusing on where you are now and what needs to be done to enhance self-care and manage secondary stress. The elements of self-care are clearly listed in the questionnaire. There may be other elements unique to your culture, personality, and lifestyle that you should include. Once you have identified the elements of your personal, self-care protocol, addressing the needs of mind, body, and spirit, we will then consider how "toxic work environments" can increase secondary stress leading burnout and influencing our attempts at self-care.

Toxic Work Environments

Designing a self-care protocol would be incomplete without some consideration of the nature of the environments in which we work, especially given that we spend more than one third of our time at work. There are two components to every work environment, the physical/structural and the cultural/psychological. Coldwell[11] describes a source of workplace stress that has evolved because of rapid developments in information technology, or what is termed the Fourth Industrial Revolution. Elsewhere in this text we have pointed to the high demands on clinicians for increased computerized documentation of care and other processes related to care such as meeting the increasing information requirements of insurers and regulators. In many cases, the work of the clinician extends far beyond hours in direct care delivery to hours in front of the computer either at work or home. This situation has led to problems of "employee well-being and mental health evidenced in cases of withdrawals from the workplace and withdrawals from work while being at work (presenteeism) and complete burnout."[11]

In an extensive literature review, Aronsson et al.[12] documented the relationship between the nature of work environments and the potential for burnout. For example, they found that an employee's control of their own work, resulted in lower emotional exhaustion and low workplace support and resulted in increased emotional exhaustion. Workplace injustice, high workload, low reward, low supervisor support, low co-worker support, and job insecurity are also correlated with emotional exhaustion and eventually burnout.[12]

In 1859, Florence Nightingale, nurse and noted health care reformer, focused on the relationship between environment and healing. She believed that "structuring a healing environment—in which the conditions of the sick room, including fresh air, light, temperature, placement of the bed, a restful and quiet atmosphere, cleanliness along with attentive care, proper nutrition and rest—were what was needed to promote a return to health."[13pp4–5] The same principles could be applied to the physical structuring of unhealthy clinical work environments with artificial light, processed air, the buzzing of machines and equipment, and as during the COVID-19 pandemic, insufficient personal protective and patient care equipment.

With respect to the psychological/cultural aspects of work environments, McKee[14] enumerated 11 factors that foster toxicity in the workplace. They are

- The demand for speed, efficiency, fast results.
- An atmosphere that discourages speaking up or questioning policy, i.e., speaking truth to power.
- Adversarial relationships—us versus. them dynamics among staff and management or various cliques and factions.
- Negative competition.
- A disconnect between stated values and actions/decisions.
- Lack of clarity, purpose, or vision.
- An atmosphere that promotes disrespect of staff or management.
- Lack of appreciation for work well done.
- Incivility, bullying, shaming, and fear tactics.

- Inequities resulting from lack of a clear meritocracy, cronyism, or forms of discrimination.[14]

Medical and nursing professionals often practice in toxic work environments. Although McKee's factors can be generally applied to health care environments, each profession may experience a unique pattern of toxicity. Jones[15] points to hospitals as toxic environments for physicians who experience unrealistic workloads because of administrative duties created by nonphysician administrators and regulators who do not understand the nuances of care. Harsh leadership can promote workplace toxicity. "Too often . . . leaders lack the finesse required for a caring profession which then inspires others to follow suit with bad behavior."[15] Khoo, a medical doctor, also points to unrealistic performance measures, an obsessive focus on numbers, quotas and revenue rather than patient care, the absence of work–life balance, and a forum in which to discuss and resolve problems.[16]

PAs often experience invisibility and a "cog in the wheel" dynamic in work environments that leads to turnover and secondary stress. Belcher, PA-C, director of the American Academy of Physician Assistants, Center for Healthcare Leadership and Management, has enumerated six conditions to improve the cultures in which physician assistants practice.

- A recognition of PA capabilities including their scope of practice.
- Operational visibility, guaranteeing that PA's work, including documentation of their work is directly attributed to them in health records and in billing.
- Leadership opportunities at the executive level in practice environments.
- Alignment of scope of practice policies with PA responsibilities.
- Avoiding compliance risks through adherence to proper billing and reimbursement practices.
- Ensuring positive work cultures where PAs are treated with respect and valued for their contributions to patient care. It should be noted that loss of a PA after 12 to 18 months of employment is estimated to cost $250,000.[17]

Toxic work environment is a key factor contributing to high turnover rates in U.S. hospitals at 19.1 percent in 2018, 4 points above the turnover rate across all U.S. industries. Grace et al.[18] documented a similarly high rate of turnover among 252 physicians, PAs, and nurse practitioners practicing in primary care clinics in California. This turnover is directly correlated with high levels of burnout as measured by the Maslach Burnout Inventory.

The American Association of Critical Care Nurses has published standards for "Establishing and Sustaining Healthy Work Environments."[19] These standards are a response to "mounting evidence that unhealthy work environments contribute to medical errors, ineffective delivery of care, and conflict and stress among health care professionals."[19]

The AACN six critical elements of healthy work environments are as follows:

- Skilled communication that reflects respect for patients and colleagues, a focus on solutions, conflict management, and appropriate communication technologies.
- True collaboration within and across clinical disciplines and with leadership.
- Effective decision making that incorporates all voices and perspectives and emphasizes accountability for collaboration.
- Appropriate staffing that considers patient acuity and staff competencies.
- Meaningful recognition including formal acknowledgement of work well done and opportunity for advancement.
- Authentic leadership that respects staff and garners the resources necessary for continued staff development.

These standards are applicable to all clinical work environments. They address not only the needs of staff but also the promotion of excellent and safe patient care, which, in the final analysis, is the goal of all medical and nursing professionals.

What will be the effect of the COVID-19 pandemic on medical and nursing professionals? Will the realities of the pandemic precipitate retirements, exits from clinical care, or difficulties in recruiting new medical and nursing professionals? What lessons will health care systems have learned about nurturing and protecting their clinicians? Will the medical and nursing professional workforce be sufficient to care for an aging, more chronically ill population in the coming decades or for a resurgence of COVID-19 or new pandemics? Recapturing the joy of clinical work through personal self-care and creating healthier work environments is crucial to the future of health care.

Self-Care and Toxic Work Environments: The Interface

Developing one's personal self-care protocol will heighten awareness of toxic factors in work environments that cause stress. Practicing self-care and knowing the characteristics of toxic work environments can be a powerful combination in preventing secondary stress and burnout. Focusing on self-care provides a renewed sense of self so that we can be healthy and flexible enough to assess and deal with constantly changing environments and determine our best person-environment fit, even if it means "moving on," or changing positions in the case of extreme work environment toxicity. As Confucius reminds us, "The way out (*may be*) through the door."

This chapter has provided a format for a designing a personal self-care protocol and a guide for assessing work environments that can be used as a springboard for supporting, challenging and creating perspective as you continue on the path of one of the most demanding and rewarding careers one can have: *health care.* We need to break our self-imposed silence concerning our need for self-care and for healthy work environments and remember that.

> Our lives begin to end the day we become silent about things that matter.
>
> —Martin Luther King Jr.

References

1. Schaufeli, WB, Bakker AB, van der Heigden FMMA, Prins JT. Workaholism among medical residents: it is the combination of working excessively and compulsively that counts. *International Journal of Stress Management.* 2009;16(R):249–272.

2. Gabbard G, Menninger R. *Medical Marriages.* Washington, DC: American Psychiatric Press; 1998.

3. Essary AC, Bernard KS, Coplan B, et al. Burnout and job and career satisfaction in the physician assistant: a review of the literature.

perspectives: *National Academy of Medicine.* https://nam.edu/wp-content/uploads/2018/11/Burnout-and-Satisfaction-in-the-PA-Profession.pdf. Published December 3, 2018. Accessed 6/17/2020.

4. Schou Andreassen C, Pallesen S, Moen BE, Bjorvatin B, Wange S, Schaufeli B. Workaholism and negative work-related incidents among nurses. *Industrial Health.* 2018 Oct 3; ;56 (5):373–381.

5. Dzau VJ, Kirch K, Nasca T. Preventing a parallel pandemic—a national strategy to protect clinicians' well-being. *New England Journal of Medicine Perspective.* 2020;383:513–515.

6. Wicks R. *Riding the Dragon.* Notre Dame, IN: Sorin Books; 2003.

7. Baker E. *Caring for Ourselves.* Washington, DC: American Psychological Association; 2001.

8. Eanes B, Richmond L, Link J. *What Brings You to Life?* Mahwah, NJ: Paulist Press; 2003.

9. Dalai Lama. *The Path to Tranquility.* New York, NY: Viking; 1999.

10. Domar A, Dreher H. *Self-Nurture.* New York, NY: Penguin Books; 2000.

11. Coldwell DAL. Negative influences of the 4th Industrial Revolution on the workplace. *International Journal of Environmental Research in Public Health.* 2019;16(15):2670.

12. Aronsson G, Theorell T, Grape T, et al. A systematic review including meta-analysis of work environment and burnout symptoms. *BMS Public Health.* 2017;17(1):264. https://pubmed.ncbi.nlm.nih.gov/28302088/ (Accessed, 6/10/2020)

13. Kennedy MS. Reflections on Nightingale's message. In: F. Nightingale, *Notes on Nursing: What It Is, and What It Is Not.* 160th Anniversary ed. Philadelphia, PA: Wolters Kluwer; 2020.

14. McKee A. *How to Be Happy at Work.* Boston, MA: Harvard Business School Publishing; 2017.

15. Jones V. What creates a toxic hospital culture? *MedPage Today's, KevinMD. com,* https://www.kevinmd.com/blog/2015/10/what-creates-a-toxic-hospital-culture.html. Published October 28, 2015. Accessed June 11, 2020.

16. Khoo R. Is your hospital a miserable place to work? here are 14 clues. *MedPage Today's, KevinMD.com,* https://www.kevinmd.com/blog/2015/09/is-your-hospital-a-miserable-place-to-work-here-are-14-clues.html. Published September 10, 2015. Accessed, 6, 11, 2020.

17. Belcher B. What PA's Want in the workplace: a supportive work environment. *American Academy of Physician Assistants, Center for Healthcare Leadership and Management.* https://www.aapa.org/news-central/2019/01/pas-want-workplace-supportive-work-environment. Published January 2019. Accessed June 11, 2020.

18. Willard-Grace R, Knox M, Huang B, Hammer H, Kivlahan C, Grumbach K. Burnout and health care workforce turnover. *Annals of Family Medicine.* 2019;17(1):36–41.

19. American Association of Critical Care Nursing. *AACN Standards for Establishing and Sustaining Healthy Work Environments.* 2nd ed. Aliso Viejo, CA: AACN; 2016.

Passionate Journeys

Returning to the Wonders of Medical and Nursing Practice

> *In dealing with those who are undergoing great suffering, if you feel "burnout" setting in, if you feel demoralized and exhausted, it is best, for the sake of everyone, to withdraw and restore yourself. The point is to have a long-term perspective.*

> —Dalai Lama

The goal of this book has been to provide information, encouragement, and direction to respect the real dangers incurred to one's psychological and physical health in the process of fulfilling the mission of practicing as a health care professional.

With the onset of Covid-19, and its immediate aftermath, medical and nursing professionals have often felt a combination of guilt, anxiety, fear, and helplessness. Long hours, lack of protective equipment, hospital overcrowding, uncertainty about the coronavirus, and the dangers of exposing self and families have created enormous stress. Through it all and against great odds, they have acted with courage and self-sacrifice closely allied with experiences that others have had during periods of protracted war. However, most physicians, nurses, and physician assistants, even under circumstances of battle fatigue, have never been required to face such acute challenges simultaneously at the bedside and at home.

Also, like the experience of posttraumatic stress disorder, it may seem like the stress never ends. In interviewing critical care nurses, it is not unusual to hear under "normal circumstances" that they later ruminate over activities during their shift. "Did I give the right dose of the medication to that young person? Did I check the wristband for allergies to medications? Was I distracted by the code that happened earlier? Should I have called the family sooner when the patient started to decline?

During prolonged and sometimes mandatory overtime hours, many spent by health care providers during the COVID-19 pandemic's height, the ruminating became even worse for some—they couldn't stop thinking about what they had done; in colloquial terms: they couldn't turn their brain off to what had happened.

Compounding the problem is that because of COVID-19's contagion, the nurse, physician assistant, physician, or other healthcare professional winds up being the "loved one" physically present, although someone from the family may be "there" electronically as is described in the following May 17, 2020 *New York Times* first page story by Jan Hoffman:

> The coronavirus patient, a 75-year-old man was dying. No family member was allowed in the room with him, only a young nurse.
>
> In full protective hear, she dimmed the lights and put on quiet music. She freshened his pillows, dabbed his lips with moistened swabs, held his hand spoke softly to him. He wasn't even her patient, but everyone else was slammed.
>
> Finally, she held an iPad close to him, so he could see the face and hear the voice of a grief-stricken relative Skyping from the hospital corridor.
>
> After the man died, the nurse found a secluded hallway, and wept.[1p1]

Much of this acute stress exacerbates the chronic pressures evident in modern health care today. And so, monitoring one's own personal well-being is not a nicety for the current caregiver—it is a *necessity*.

Moreover, in addition to the personal benefits derived from self-care, how the health care professional addresses this area can have a beneficial impact on those being served. It is no surprise that unfortunate—and sometimes even fatal—consequences for innocent patients may be attributable to the inattentiveness and exhaustion of harried, hurried health care personnel who ignore or minimize the value of both self-care and self-knowledge.

Christensen and Suchman summarize the realistic strains of modern health care:

> Caring for the health of human beings is a vocation that has summoned forth some of the noblest and most valued work in human societies through the millennia. . . . With increased integration of services, constraints on society's financing

of health care, a swelling of the population moving into advanced age, and the acceleration of information processing technologies—increased demands are falling on the backs of professionals throughout the healthcare spectrum for increased productivity, documentation, vigilance to prevent error, and mastery of expanding areas of knowledge and technology. We often find ourselves racing to keep up with all our tasks without having time to reflect on the deeper meaning of our vocation. The load we are carrying increasingly exceeds our carrying capacity.[2p2]

Yet even though the stresses and strains can be extreme, the theme and philosophical stance of their message highlights that *recapturing the awe of being a physician, nurse, or physician's assistant is within reach with some knowledge and action.* What is almost lost can be rediscovered. What is presently possessed need not be given away. A recently graduated nurse at a leading teaching hospital shared how much joy her work was bringing her. In doing this, she then described some of her cases and challenges, as well as her frustrations. Chief among her complaints was that some of her co-workers in the intensive care unit seemed drained, jaded, and unmotivated. She said in a hoarse voice, "I don't want to get that way. Nursing is a gift I don't want to lose or take for granted." Our point in writing the revision of this book is that this nurse, or any health professional for that matter, does not have to succumb to the stresses of work like her co-workers.

Furthermore, during a pandemic (as in the case of other crises), the possibility for the physician, physician assistant, or nurse to experience posttraumatic growth also becomes more of a reality, although it is by no means, guaranteed—especially if two elements in one's outlook are not embraced: *clarity and openness.* On the one hand, during a dark period in one's life, one must be clear about the trauma or serious stress one is facing. Denying, avoiding, diminishing, or romanticizing what one is encountering is not helpful. On the other hand, not being open to where this unwanted, negative experience might lead is also problematic since it may deny one the discovery of new personal depth or an appreciation of a greater quality of life.

No one wants a crisis or an encounter with personal darkness. Yet, if such a trauma or period of serious stress and life disruption does take place and we have no choice about it, we still have a possibility to grow (and this is important to note) *in ways that would not have been possible had the trauma or darkness not occurred in the first place.*

This book then has been about retaining and deepening the gift of passion for the care of others while realistically facing the interior and systemic acute and chronic problems that are part of an involved life—especially in such personally and intellectually demanding fields as medicine and nursing. It has also dealt with having a real sensitivity to the acute and chronic dangers to one's health while not consequently forsaking the honor and privilege of working in health care.

Equally important, this work has been about diagnosing the problems of *secondary* stress early, taking action—both preventive and ameliorative—as soon as possible, and reviewing the results of such ongoing interventions. To do this, one needs to be aware of what can be learned from the literature on the topic and from clinical work. Above all, it is about coming home to oneself in a way that self-knowledge, strengthening one's inner life, and self-care are not considered "a given" or "a luxury" but are instead intentionally embraced as part of an essential ongoing process. Such a process, like effective therapy, produces good results and a return to the wonder and awe that entering and remaining in the medical and nursing health fields can and should produce.

There is a need for an ongoing monitoring of oneself and a continual posing of questions such as the following:

- What approaches are most helpful for me to take to deal with the systemic and personal stresses in healthcare and in my life now?
- What additional knowledge/support do I need to take actions to accomplish a better program of self-care and increased self-knowledge?
- How can I become more resilient both personally and professionally as well as enhance the healthcare system within which I am currently working?

In the previous five chapters, we enumerated the many benefits of facing these questions in a conscious, ongoing (sometimes formal) way. To review, some of the primary benefits may include

- An ability to focus on the patient in front of you—no matter how full your day may be.
- A sense of intrigue about your talents and growing edges in ways that help you deepen your professional and personal life.

- A willingness and facility to appropriately handle strong emotions, deal with different patients/colleagues, clarify roles, and improve your level of satisfaction in interpersonal relations.
- A recognition of the need for time apart to reflect, reassess, and replenish yourself.
- A willingness to speak up, directly and respectfully, in difficult situations with the goal of improving the care of patients and environments of care.
- Awareness of the signs of chronic irritability, fatigue, constant daydreaming, greater effort with lesser job satisfaction, inability to relax, and a tendency to be preoccupied with work as warnings that chronic secondary stress needs to be limited before it becomes too severe.

This book is designed to keep close at hand for quick reference. Open it often, underline passages that resonate with you, mark the pages, write in the margins, Delving into the text and examining your responses to the questionnaires will enable you to tailor your approach to and efforts at self-care.

The Joys of Medicine and Nursing

As one takes reasonable steps toward facing the challenges of *secondary* stress, to retain a sense of perspective there is also a need to recall the joys of being a professional in health care today. Too often we focus on just the dangers, challenges, and stress, and we fail to recall the joys. Being a medical or nursing professional is very rewarding in so many ways. These include

- Saving, improving, or prolonging people's lives.
- Receiving trust and being part of the dramatic elements of peoples' lives not open to many other people/professionals.
- Being part of a profession, whose knowledge base is dynamic and deep.
- Having the security of knowing that medical/nursing professionals will always be needed and valued.
- Experiencing a sense of potency because of the impact you may have on other peoples' lives.

- Influencing the way in which care is delivered in health care settings and communities.
- Having opportunities to interact with a wide range of people and emotions in a myriad of situations.
- Being able to be both intrigued and challenged by the resistance of a disease (and sometimes the person carrying it!) to the treatment protocol you provide.
- Knowing first-hand the benefit of both good organization and creativity in providing sound interventions—and the challenges that lie in knowing when one takes precedent over the other.
- Appreciating the essential role your own personality, spirituality, and psychological health has in delivering effective health care.
- Having the chance to be a "detective" as you seek to uncover the meaning of symptoms and signs as you track and/or unmask a previously undiagnosed/undetected disease or illness in a patient or predisposing environmental situations.

The joys of clinical work can be so great. However, as in the case of self-care, they are not a given. They must be appreciated and attended to in our lives. When faced with stress, medical and nursing professionals all act. The question this book confronts is: How do we act? If we do not develop careful strategies, either inactivity or unhealthy actions will certainly fill the void. It is our hope in writing the revision of this book that the reader will set aside resistance to understanding, limiting, and overcoming secondary stress. After reading this book, using the questionnaires and tables as follow-up, and revisiting the book when issues re-emerge—and they will—we believe that practitioners will navigate the waves of stress that come in health care in the most healthy way possible. Moreover, the result of such experiences will open the medical and nursing professional to be a deeper person and a helpful mentor to colleagues and students who, like them, give much and deserve all the support and wisdom we can share.

References

1.   Hoffman J. I can't turn my brain off: PTSD and burnout threaten medical workers. *New York Times,* May 17, 2020, p. 1.
2.   Christensen J, Suchman A. Introduction. *Medical Encounter.* 2002;16(4) 2.

Bibliography

Accreditation Review Commission on Education for the Physician Assistant, Inc. *Accreditation Standards for Physician Assistant Education*. Johns Creek, GA: ARC-PA; 2019.

Accreditation Review Commission on Education for the Physician Assistant, Inc. *Standards for Physician Assistant Education*. 5th ed. http://www.arc-pa.org/wp-content/uploads/2020/07/AccredManual-5th-ed-7.20.pdf. Published July 2020. Accessed August 27, 2020.

Aitken, R. *The Mind of Clover: Essays on Zen Buddhist Ethics*. San Francisco, CA: North Point Press; 1984.

American Association of Critical Care Nursing. *AACN Standards for Establishing and Sustaining Healthy Work Environments*. 2nd ed. Aliso Viejo, CA: AACN; 2016.

Ammerman RT, Cassisi JE, Hersen M, Van-Hasselt VB. Consequences of physical abuse and neglect in children. *Clinical Psychology Review*. 1986;6:291–310.

Aronsson G, Theorell T, Grape T, et al. A systematic review including meta-analysis of work environment and burnout symptoms. *BMS Public Health*. 2017;17(1):264.

Auden WH. *Introduction to Dag Hammarskjold's* Markings. New York: Knopf; 1976.

Baez J. Merton the prophet. In: Wilkes P, ed. *Merton: By Those Who Knew Him Best* San Francisco, CA: Harper; 1984: 41–46.

Bailey R, Clarke M. *Stress and Coping in Nursing*. New York, NY: Chapman and Hall; 1989.

Baker E. *Caring for Ourselves: A Therapist's Guide to Personal and Professional Well-being*. Washington, DC: American Psychological Association; 2003.

Barnum B. *Spirituality in Nursing*. 2nd ed: *From Traditional to New Age*. New York: Springer; 2003.

Beck DF. Counselor burnout in family service agencies. *Social Casework*. 1987;68(1):3–15.

Belcher B. What PA's want in the workplace: a supportive work environment. *American Academy of Physician Assistants*. https://www.aapa.org/news-central/2019/01/pas-want-workplace-supportive-work-environment/. Published January 2019. Accessed June 11, 2020.

Ben-Sira Z. Stress and illness: a revised application of the stressful life events approach research communications in psychology. *Psychiatry and Behavior*. 1981;6:317–327.

Benson H. *Timeless Healing: The Power and Biology of Beliefs*. New York, NY: Charles Scribner; 1996.

Bentley J, Toth M. *Exploring Wicked Problems: What They Are and Why They Are Important*. Bloomington, IN: Archway; 2020.

Block D. Foreword. In: Scott C, Hawk J, eds. *Heal Thyself: The Health of Health Care Professionals*. New York, NY: Brunner Mazel; 1986: ix.

Bloom A. *Beginning to Pray*. Ramsey, NJ: Paulist Press; 1970.

Bode R. *First You Have to Row a Little Boat*. New York, NY: Warner, 1993.

Bond M. *Stress and Self-Awareness: A Guide for Nurses*. Rockville, MD: Aspen; 1986.

Brazier D. *Zen Therapy*. New York, NY: Wiley; 1995.

Briere J. *Therapy for Adults Molested as Children: Beyond Survival*. New York, NY: Springer; 1989.

Buber M. *Way of Man*. New York, NY: Lyle Stuart; 1966.

Burns D. *Feeling Good*. New York, NY: Thomas More/Sorin Books; 2000.

Byrd R. *Alone*. New York: Kodansha; 1995. Original work published 1938.

Carpenter H. ANA's health risk appraisal: three years later. *American Nurse Today*. https://www.myamericannurse.com/wp-content/uploads/2016/12/ant1-NPWE-1219.pdf. Published January 2017. Accessed 6/18/2020.

Castaneda C. *Journey to Ixilan: The Lessons of Don Juan*. New York, NY: Simon and Schuster; 1972.

Center for Disease Control and Prevention. Estimated influenza illnesses, medical visits, hospitalizations, and deaths in the US 2018–19 influenza season. https://www.cdc.gov/flu/about/burden/2018-2019.html. Published January 8, 2020. Accessed May 11, 2020.

Ceslowitz SB. Burnout and coping strategies among hospital staff nurses. *Journal of Advanced Nursing*. 1989;14:553–558.

Chadwick D. *The Crooked Cucumber*. New York, NY: Broadway; 1999.

Cherniss C. *Beyond Burnout*. New York, NY: Routledge; 1995.

Chodron P. *When Things Fall Apart*. Boston, MA: Shambala; 1997.

Christensen J, Suchman A. Introduction. *Medical Encounter*. 2002;16(4):2.

Coldwell DAI. Negative influences of the 4th Industrial Revolution on the workplace. *International Journal of Environmental Research in Public Health.* 2019;16(15):2670.

Conklin J. Wicked problems and social complexity, 2001–2005. Cognexus Institute. https://cognexus.org/wpf/wickedproblems.pdf. Accessed 6/10/2020.

Coombs R, Fawzy F. The impaired-physician syndrome: a developmental perspective. In: Scott C, Hawk J, eds. *Heal Thyself.* New York, NY: Brunner/Mazel; 1986.

Coplan B, McCall TC, Smith M, Gellert VL, Essary AC. Burnout, job satisfaction and stress levels of Physician Assistants. *Journal of the American Academy of Physician Assistants.* 2018;31(9):42–46.

Coster J, Schwebel M. Well-functioning in professional psychologists. *Professional Psychology: Research and Practice.* 1997;28:5–13.

Cousins N., *Anatomy of an Illness as Perceived by the Patient.* New York, NY: W. W. Norton; 1979.

Dalai Lama. *The Path to Tranquility.* New York, NY: Penguin; 2000.

De Chant P, Shannon DW. *Preventing Physician Burnout: A Handbook for Physicians and Health Care Leaders.* North Charleston, SC: Simpler Healthcare; 2016.

Domar A, Dreher H. *Self-Nurture: Learning to Care for Yourself as Effectively as You Care for Everyone Else.* New York, NY: Penguin; 2000.

Donnelly G. *Coping With Stress: RN's Survival Sourcebook.* Oradell, NJ: Medical Economics Company; 1983.

Donnelly, G. Pandemic: looking back and thinking ahead. *Holistic Nursing Practice.* 2020;34(4):93–94.

Dubois D. Renewal of prayer. *Lumen Vitae.* 1983;38(3):273–274.

Dyrbye, LN, Thomas MR, Huntington JL, et al. Personal life events and medical student burnout: a multicenter study. *Academic Medicine.* 2006;81:374–384.

Dzau VJ, Kirch K, Nasca T. Preventing a parallel pandemic—a national strategy to protect clinicians' well-being. *New England Journal of Medicine Perspective.* 2020;383:513–515.

e.e. cummings. Unpublished letter to a high school editor; 1955.

Eanes B, Richmond L, Link J. *What Brings You to Life: Awakening Spiritual Essence.* Mahwah, NJ: Paulist Press; 2001.

Edelwich J, Brodsky A. *Burnout.* New York, NY: Human Sciences Press; 1980.

Eiser A. *The Ethos of Medicine in Post Modern America.* Lanham, MD: Lexington Books; 2014.

Emory N. Tracking the mind–body connection: an interview with Herbert Benson. *Brain World.* https://brainworldmagazine.com/tracking-mind-body-connection-interview-dr-herbert-benson/. November 7, 2019. Accessed June 2, 2020.

Enders LE, Mercier JM. Treating chemical dependency: the need for including the family. *International Journal of Addictions.* 1993;28:507–519.

Epictetus. *The Art of Living.* Sharon Lebell, ed. New York, NY: Harper One; 1995.

Epictetus. *The Enchiridion.* http://classics.mit.edu/Epictetus/epicench.html. Accessed May 14, 2020. Original work published 135 BCE.

Epstein LC, Thomas CB, Shaffer JW, Perlin S. Clinical prediction of physician suicide based on medical student data. *Journal of Nervous and Mental Disease.* 1973;156:19–29.

Essary AC, Bernard KS, Coplan B, et al. Burnout and job and career satisfaction in the physician assistant: a review of the literature. *Perspectives: National Academy of Medicine.* https://nam.edu/wp-content/uploads/2018/11/ Burnout-and-Satisfaction-in-the-PA-Profession.pdf. Published December 3, 2018. Accessed 6/17//2020.

Figley C. ed. *Treating Compassion Fatigue.* New York, NY: Brunner-Routledge; 2002.

Figley C, Huggard P, Rees CE. *First Do No Self-Harm: Understanding and Promoting Physician Stress Resilience.* New York, NY: Oxford University Press; 2013.

Fimian MJ, Fastenau PS, Thomas J. Stress in nursing and intentions to leave the profession. *Psychological Reports.* 1989;62:105–111.

Firth H, Britton P. "Burnout," Absence, and turnover amongst British nursing staff. *Journal of Occupational Psychology.* 1989;62:55–59.

Flach F. *Putting the Pieces Together Again: A Physician's Guide to Thriving on Stress.* New York, NY: Hatherleigh Press.

Foa EB, Steketee G, Olasov Rothbaum B. Behavioral/cognitive conceptualizations of post-traumatic stress disorder. *Behavior Therapy.* 1989;20:155–176.

Foy DW, Drescher K, Fitz A, Kennedy K. Post Traumatic Stress Disorders. In: Wicks R, Parsons R, Capps D, eds. *Clinical Handbook of Pastoral Counseling.* Vol. 3. Mahwah, NJ: Paulist Press; 2003: 274–288.

Foy DW, Osato S, Houskamp B, Neumann D. Etiology factors in posttraumatic stress disorder. In: Saigh P, ed. *Posttraumatic Stress Disorder: A Behavioral Approach to Assessment and Treatment.* Oxford, UK: Pergamon Press; 1992: 28–49.

Foy DW, Sipprelle RC, Rueger DB, Carroll EM. Etiology of posttraumatic stress disorder in Vietnam veterans: analysis of pre-military, military, and combat exposure influences. *Journal of Consulting and Clinical Psychology.* 1984;52:79–87.

Frank E. Self-care, prevention, and health promotion. In: Goldman LS, Myers M, Dickstein LJ, eds. *The Handbook of Physician Health.* Chicago, IL: American Medical Association, 2000.

Freudenberger H. Impaired clinicians: coping with burnout. In: Keller PA, Ritt L, eds. *Innovations in Clinical Practice: A Sourcebook*. Vol 3. Sarasota, FL: Professional Resource Exchange; 1984: 221–228.

Freudenberger HJ. The health professional in treatment: symptoms, dynamics, and treatment issues. In: Scott CD, Hawk J, eds. *Heal Thyself: The Health of Health Care Professionals*. New York, NY: Brunner Mazel; 1986: 185–193.

Freudenberger HJ, North G. *Women's Burnout: How to Spot It, How to Reverse It, and How to Prevent It*. Garden City, NY: Doubleday; 1985.

Gilbert D. *Stumbling on Happiness*. New York, NY: Knopf; 2006.

Gill J. Burnout: a growing threat to ministry. *Human Development*. 1980;1(2):21–27.

Goodwin JM, Goodwin JS, Kellner R. Psychiatric symptoms in disliked medical patients. *Journal of American Medical Association*. 1979;241:1117–1120.

Gorky M. *Gorky: My Childhood*. London: Penguin; 1996.

Gray-Toft P, Anderson JG. The Nursing Stress Scale: development of an instrument. *Journal of Behavioral Assessment*. 1981;3:117–123.

Green BL, Grace MC, Gleser GC. Identifying survivors at risk: long-term impairment following the Beverly Hills Supper Club fire. *Journal of Clinical and Consulting Psychology*. 1985;53(185):672–678.

Gunderson L. Physician burnout. *Annals of Internal Medicine*. 2001;135:145–148.

Halbesleben JRB, Rothert C. Linking physician burnout and patient outcomes: exploring the dyadic relationships between physicians and patients. *Health Care Management Review*. 2008;33(1):29–39.

Hallet PE. *The English Pyryers of St. Thomas More Written when He Was a Prisoner in the Tower of London in 1534*. West Conshocken, PA: Templeton Publishers, 1995.

Hanh, TN. *No Mud, No Lotus: The Art of Transforming Suffering*. Berkeley, CA: Parallax Press; 2014.

Helm D. The healthy building movement: a focus on occupants. *Floor Daily*. https://www.floordaily.net/floorfocus/the-healthy-building-movement-a-focus-on-occupants-augsep-2017. Published May 14, 2020. Accessed May 14, 2020.

Heschel A. *The Insecurity of Freedom*. New York, NY: Farrar, Straus, and Giroux; 1951.

Heschel A. On prayer. *Conservative Judaism*. 1970;25(1):1–12.

Hood R, Spilka B, Budsberger B, Gorsuch R. *The Psychology of Religion*. New York, NY: Guilford Press; 1986.

Houskamp BM, Foy DW. The assessment of posttraumatic stress disorder in battered women. *Journal of Interpersonal Violence*. 1991;6:367–375.

Jacobson SF, McGrath HM, eds. *Nurses Under Stress*. New York, NY: Wiley; 1983.

Johnston-Taylor E. *Fast Facts About Religion for Nurses: Implications for Patient Care*. New York, NY: Springer; 2019.

Jones V. What creates a toxic hospital culture? October 28, 2015, *MedPage Today's KevinMD.com*. https://www.kevinmd.com/blog/2015/10/what-creates-a-toxic-hospital-culture.html. Published October 2015. Accessed June 11, 2020.

Kaplan A. *Meditation and Kabbalah*. York Beach, ME: Samuel Weiser; 1982.

Keane TM, Fairbank JA, Caddell JM, Zimering RT. Therapy reduces symptoms of PTSD in Vietnam combat veterans. *Behavior Therapy*. 1989;20:245–260.

Kennedy MS. Reflections on Nightingales message. In Nightingale F, ed. *Notes on Nursing: What It Is, and What It Is Not*. 160th anniversary ed. Philadelphia, PA: Wolters Kluwer; 2020: 4–5.

Khoo R. Is your hospital a miserable place to work? Here are 14 clues. *MedPage Today's KevinMD.com*. https://www.kevinmd.com/blog/2015/09/is-your-hospital-a-miserable-place-to-work-here-are-14-clues.html. Published September 10, 2015. Accessed June 11, 2020.

Koenig HG. *Religion, spirituality and health: the research and clinical implications. International Scholarly Research Network Psychiatry*. 2012;2012:1–3.

Kolb LC. A critical survey of hypotheses regarding posttraumatic stress disorders in light of recent research findings. *Journal of Traumatic Stress*. 1988;1(3):291–304.

Kornfield J. *A Path With Heart*. New York, NY: Bantam; 1993.

Kottler J. *On Being a Therapist*. San Francisco, CA: Jossey-Bass; 1986.

Kupferschmidt K. The coronavirus czar. *Science*. 2020;368(6490):462–465.

Kupferschmidt K. The lockdown worked—but what comes next. *Science*. 2020;368(6488):218–219.

Lachman VD. *Stress Management: A Manual for Nurses*. New York, NY: Grune and Stratton; 1983.

Lazarus RS, Folkman S. *Stress, Appraisal, and Coping*. New York, NY: Springer; 1984.

Leech K. *Soul Friend*. San Francisco, CA: Harper and Row; 1980.

Leigh H, Reiser F. *The Patient*. New York: Plenum Press; 1980.

Luo H, Galasso A. The one good thing caused by COVID-19: innovation. *Working Knowledge: Harvard Business School* https://hbswk.hbs.edu/item/the-one-good-thing-caused-by-covid-19-innovation. Published May 7, 2020. Accessed May 12, 2020.

Martin J. *Between Heaven and Mirth: When Joy, Humor and Laughter Are at the Heart of Spiritual Life*. New York, NY: Harper Collins; 2011.

Maslach C. Burned-out. *Human Behavior*. 1976;5:16–22.

Maslach C. *Burnout: The Cost of Caring*. New York, NY: Prentice-Hall; 1982.

Maslach C. Job burnout: how people cope. *Public Welfare*. 1978;36(2):56–58.

McCaffrey R, Fairbank J. Behavioral assessment and treatment of accident-related posttraumatic stress disorder: two case studies. *Behavior Therapy*. 1985;16:406–416.

McConnel E. *Burnout in the Nursing Profession.* St. Louis, MO: Mosby; 1982.

McKee A. *How to Be Happy at Work.* Boston, MA: Harvard Business School; 2017.

Mee CL. Battling burnout. *Nursing.* 2002;32(8):8.

Mentink J, Scott CD. Implementing a self-care curriculum. In: Scott CD, Hawk J, eds. *Heal Thyself: The Health of Health Care Professionals.* New York, NY: Brunner Mazel; 1986: 235–256.

Merton T. *A Vow of Conversation.* New York, NY: Farrar, Straus, and Giroux; 1988.

Miller M, Fry WF. The effect of mirthful laughter on the human cardiovascular system. *Medical Hypotheses.* 2009;73(5):636.

Moss F, Paice E. Getting things right for the doctor in training. In: Firth Cozens J, Payne R, eds. *Stress in Health Professionals: Psychological and Organizational Causes and Interventions.* New York, NY: Wiley; 1999: 203–218.

Muldasy T. *Burnout and Health Professionals: Manifestations and Management.* Norwalk, CT: Appleton-Century-Crofts; 1983.

Myers M, Dickstein LJ, eds. *The Handbook of Physician Health.* Chicago, IL: American Medical Association; 2000.

Nesse R. A wicked problem: health care system reform and change. *Council of Accountable Physician Practices.* https://accountablecaredoctors.org/health-care-reform/a-wicked-problem-healthcare-system-reform-and-change/. Published 2009. Accessed Mary 9, 2020.

Nouwen H. *Making All Things New.* New York, NY: Harper and Row; 1981.

Nouwen H. *The Way of the Heart.* New York, NY: Seabury/Harper Collins; 1981.

Novack DH, Suchman AL, Clark W, et al. Calibrating the physician: personal awareness and effective patient care. *Journal of American Medical Association.* 1997;278(6):502–509.

O'Brien M. *Spirituality in Nursing: Standing on Holy Ground.* 2nd ed. Boston, MA: Jones and Bartlett; 2003.

Pargament K. *The Psychology of Religion and Coping.* New York, NY: Guilford Press; 1997.

Pargament K. Religious methods of coping: resources for conservation and transformation of significance. In Shafranske EP, ed. *Religion and the Clinical Practice of Psychology.* Washington, DC: American Psychiatric Association; 1996: Chapter 8.

Payne N. Occupational stressors and coping as determinants of burnout in female hospice nurses. *Journal of Advanced Nursing.* 2001;33:396–406.

Peterson T. Health in America is a wicked problem. *Stakeholder Health.* https://stakeholderhealth.org/wicked-problem/. Published January 20, 2016. Accessed May 12, 2020.

Pfifferling JH. Coping with residency distress. *Resident and Staff Physician.* 1983;29:105–111.

Pfifferling JH. Cultural antecedents promoting professional impairment. In Scott CD, Hawk J, eds. *Heal Thyself: The Health of Healthcare Professionals.* New York, NY: Brunner Mazel; 1986: 3–18.

Pfifferling JH. Managing the unmanageable: the disruptive physician. *Family Practice Management.* 1997;4(10):76–92.

Pines AM, Aronson E, Kafry D. *Burnout: From Tedium to Personal Growth.* New York, NY: Free Press; 1981.

Provine RR. *Laughter: A Scientific Investigation.* New York, NY: Penguin Books; 2000.

Purcell JM. *A Review of the Literature on Burnout in Nurses: Implications for Prevention and Treatment.* Columbia, MO: University of Missouri Press; 1995.

Reinhold B. *Toxic Work.* New York, NY: Plume; 1997.

Rice VH, ed. *Handbook of Stress, Coping, and Health: Implications for Nursing Research, Theory, and Practice.* Thousand Oaks, CA: SAGE; 2000.

Rilke R. *Letters to a Young Poet.* New York, NY: Norton; 1954.

Rinpoche S. *The Tibetan Book of Living and Dying.* New York, NY: Harper Collins; 2002.

Rittel HWJ, Webber MM. Dilemmas in a general theory of planning. *Policy Sciences.* 1973;4:155–169.

Roberts L. Pandemic brings mass vaccinations to a halt. *Science.* 2020;368 (6487):116–117.

Rodman R. *Keeping Hope Alive.* New York, NY: Harper and Row; 1985.

Roy A. Suicide in doctors. *Psychiatric Clinics of North America.* 1985;8(2):377–387.

Salinsky J, Sacklin P. eds. *What Are You Feeling, Doctor?* Oxford, UK: Radcliffe Medical Press, 2000.

Sanders L. *The Case of Lucy Bending.* New York, NY: Putnam; 1982.

Schafer W. *Stress, Distress and Growth.* Davis, CA: Responsible Action; 1978.

Schaufeli W, Maslach C, Marek T, eds. *Professional Burnout.* Florence, KY: Taylor and Francis; 1993.

Schaufeli WB, Bakker AB, van der Heigden FMMA, Prins JT. Workaholism among medical residents: it is the combination of working excessively and compulsively that counts. *International Journal of Stress Management.* 2009;16: 249–272.

Schou Andreassen C, Pallesen S, Moen BE, Bjorvatin B, Wange S, Schaufeli B. Workaholism and negative work-related incidents among nurses. *Industrial Health.* 2018;56:373–381.

Scott C, Hawk J, eds. *Heal Thyself: The Health of Health Care Professionals.* New York, NY: Brunner Mazel; 1986.

Seligman MEP. Learned helplessness. In: Levitt E, Rubin B, Brooks J, eds. *Depression: Concepts, Controversies and Some New Facts.* Hillsdale, NJ: Erlbaum; 1983: 306–327.

Selye H. *Stress Without Distress*. Philadelphia, PA: JB Lippincott; 1974.

Sevak S, Romundstad S, Homan J. A 7-year prospective study of sense of humor and mortality in an adult county population. *International Journal of Psychiatry in Medicine*. 2010;40(2):125–146.

Seward B. *Managing Stress in Emergency Medical Services*. Sudbury, MA: American Academy of Orthopedic Surgeons, Jones, and Bartlett; 2000.

Silverman MM. Physicians and suicide. In: Goldman LS, Myers M, Dickstein LJ, eds. *The Handbook of Physician Health*. Chicago, IL: American Medical Association; 2000: 95–117.

Smythe E. *Surviving Nursing*. Los Angeles, CA: Western Schools; 1994.

Snowden, F.M. *Epidemics and Society. From the Black Death to the Present*. New Haven, CT: Yale University Press; 2019.

Sotile WM, Sotile MO. *The Medical Marriage: Sustaining Healthy Relationship for Physicians and Their Families*. Chicago, IL: American Medical Association; 2000.

Sotile WM, Sotile MO. *The Resilient Physician*. Chicago, IL: American Medical Association; 2002.

Spike J, Carlin N. Ethical decisions: stress and distress in medicine. In: Figley C, Huggard P, Rees CE, eds. *First Do No Harm: Understanding and Promoting Physician Stress Resilience*. New York, NY: Oxford University Press; 2013: 281–293.

Steindler EM. The role of professional organizations in developing support. In: Scott CD, Hawk J, eds. *Heal Thyself: The Health of Health Care Professionals*. New York, NY: Brunner Mazel; 1986: 2217–227.

Steinmetz J, Blankenship J, Brown L, et al. *Managing Stress Before It Manages You*. Palo Alto, CA: Bull; 1980.

Steinmetz J, Proctor S, Hall D, et al. *Rx for Stress: A Nurse's Guide*. Palo Alto, CA: Bull; 1984.

Storr A. *On Solitude*. New York, NY: Bantam; 1988.

Strand C. *The Wooden Bowl*. New York, NY: Hyperion; 1988.

Sullivan P, Burka L. Results from CMA's huge 1998 physician survey point to a dispirited profession. *Canadian Medical Association Journal*. 159;1998:525–529.

Summers S, Summers HJ. *Saving Lives: Why the Media's Portrayal of Nursing Puts Us All at Risk*. New York, NY: Oxford University Press; 2015.

Takakuwa K, Rubashkin N, Herzig K, eds. *What I Learned in Medical School: Personal Stories of Young Doctors*. Berkeley, CA: University of California Press; 2004.

Tate P. *The Doctor's Communication Handbook*. Oxford, UK: Radcliffe Medical Press; 2001.

Thomas S. *Transforming Nurses' Stress and Anger: Steps Toward Healing*. New York, NY: Springer; 2004.

Twain M. *The Adventures of Huckleberry Finn.* Project Guttenberg, E-Book #76, https://www.gutenberg.org/files/76/76-h/76-h.htm. Updated May 25, 2018. Original work published 1885. Accessed May 14, 2020.

Tyson, PD, Pongruengphant R, Aggarwal B. Coping with organizational stress among hospital nurses in southern Ontario. *International Journal of Nursing Studies.* 2002;39(4):453–459.

Ullrich A, FitzGerald P. Stress experienced by physicians and nurses in the cancer ward. *Social Science and Medicine.* 1990;31(9):1013–1022.

United Nations. COVID-19 and the need for action on mental health. UN Policy Brief. https://unsdg.un.org/sites/default/files/2020-05/UN-Policy-Brief-COVID-19-and-mental-health.pdf. Published May 13, 2020. Accessed August 27, 2020.

Valtorta NK, Kanaan M, Gilbody S, Hanratty B. Loneliness, social isolation and risk of cardiovascular disease in the English longitudinal study of ageing. *European Journal of Preventive Cardiology.* 2018;25(13):1389–1396.

Watzalawick P, Weakland J, Fisch R. *Change: Principles of Problem Formation and Problem Resolution.* New York, NY: W. W. Norton; 1974.

Weems C. *HA! The Science of When We Laugh and Why.* New York, NY: Basic Books; 2014.

Welles JF. *The Story of Stupidity.* Orient, NY: Mt. Pleasant Press; 1988.

Wessells D, Kutscher A, Seeland IB, Selder FE, Cherico DJ, Clark EJ, eds. *Professional Burnout in Medicine and the Helping Professions.* New York, NY: Haworth Press; 1989.

Whittington R. Attitudes toward patient aggression amongst mental health nurses in the "zero tolerance" era: associations with burnout and length of experience. *Journal of Clinical Nursing.* 2002;11:819–825.

Wicks R. *After 50: Spiritually Embracing Your Own Wisdom Years.* Mahwah, NJ: Paulist Press; 1997.

Wicks R. *Availability.* New York, NY: Crossroad; 1986.

Wicks R. Countertransference and burnout in pastoral counseling. In: Wicks R, Parsons R, Capps D, eds. *Clinical Handbook of Pastoral Counseling.* Vol. 3. Mahwah, NJ: Paulist Press; 2003: 321–341.

Wicks R. Guilt and the corona virus. *Nursing 2020.* April 2020.

Wicks R. *Living a Gentle, Passionate Life.* Mahwah, NJ: Paulist Press; 1998.

Wicks R. *Living Simply in an Anxious World.* Mahwah, NJ: Paulist Press; 1988.

Wicks R. Resilience in a time of crisis. *Nursing.* 2020;6:49–51.

Wicks R. *Riding the Dragon: 10 Lessons for Inner Strength in Challenging Times.* Notre Dame, IN: Sorin Books; 2003.

Wicks R. *Seeds of Sensitivity: Deepening Your Spiritual Life.* Notre Dame, IN: AMP; 1995.

Wicks R. *Simple Changes: Quietly Overcoming Barriers to Personal and Professional Growth.* Allen, TX: Thomas More; 2000.

Wicks R. The stress of spiritual ministry: practical suggestions on avoiding unnecessary distress. In: Wicks R, ed. *Handbook of Spirituality for Ministers*, Vol. 1. Mahwah, NJ: Paulist Press; 1995: 249–258.

Wicks R. *Touching the Holy: Ordinariness, Self-Esteem, and Friendship*. Notre Dame, IN: Ave Maria Press; 1992.

Wicks R, Hamma R. *Circle of Friends*. Notre Dame, IN: AMP, 1996.

Wicks R, Parsons R, Capps D. *Clinical Handbook of Pastoral Counseling*, Vol. 3. Mahwah, NJ: Paulist Press; 2003.

Williams E, Konrad T, Scheckler W, et al. Understanding physicians' intentions to withdraw from practice: the role of job satisfaction, job stress, and mental and physical health. *Health Care Management Review*. 2001;26(1):7–19.

Wolfe G. Burnout of therapists. *Physical Therapy*. 1981;61:10467–1050.

Yam BMC, Shiu ATY. Perceived stress and sense of coherence among critical care nurses in Hong Kong: a pilot study. *Journal of Clinical Nursing*. 2003;12:144–147.

Yao DC, Wright SM. National survey of internal medicine residency program directors regarding problem residents. *Journal of American Medical Association*. 2000;284(9):1099–1104.

Websites

The following websites are useful in accessing the most current information on the concepts and management of stress, secondary stress, burnout, PTSD, toxic work environments and self-care, including also, specific pages of the major professional associations on these issues.

Physician Websites

AMA Continuing Education programs to enhance professional well-being. https://edhub.ama-assn.org/steps-forward/pages/professional-well-being

AMA's Joy in Medicine program https://edhub.ama-assn.org/steps-forward/module/2702510

Burnout medical residents https://www.ama-assn.org/residents-students/resident-student-health/burnout-medical-residents-unearthing-bigger-picture

Physician Assistant Websites

The American Academy of Physician Assistants https://www.aapa.org/news-central/2019/01/pas-want-workplace-supportive-work-environment/

Burnout among Rural Physician Assistants https://journals.lww.com/jpae/Abstract/2016/06000/Burnout_in_Rural_Physician_Assistants__An_Initial.7.aspx

Journal of the American Academy of Physician Assistant's study on stress among PAs https://journals.lww.com/jaapa/Fulltext/2018/09000/Burnout,_job_satisfaction,_and_stress_levels_of.8.aspx

The Physician Assistant Life https://www.thepalife.com/the-physician-assistant-physician-relationship-5-must-haves/

Nursing Websites

Bibliography on secondary stress https://www.psychiatricnursing.org/article/S0883-9417(10)00058-0/fulltext

Healthy Work Environment criteria by the American Nurses Association https://www.nursingworld.org/practice-policy/work-environment/

Nursing World Health Organization State of World Nursing https://apps.who.int/nhwaportal/Sown/Files?name=usa.pdf

Statistics on Work-Place Violence Affecting Nurses https://www.nursingworld.org/practice-policy/work-environment/end-nurse-abuse/

Hospital Trends

Beckers Hospital Review is a free listserv that reports trends in healthcare affecting hospitals https://www.beckershospitalreview.com/

Strategies to Combat Secondary Stress and Burnout

The Cochrane Library publishes and rates evidence-based research in the health fields. This site lists psychological interventions for resilience in adults https://www.cochranelibrary.com/cdsr/doi/10.1002/14651858.CD012527/full

Differentiating Burnout and Compassion Fatigue https://extinguishburnout.com/2019/08/19/is-it-compassion-fatigue-or-burnout/

Humor, Laughter and Spirituality https://www.guideposts.org/inspiration/miracles/gods-grace/divine-humor-how-laughter-benefits-us-spiritually

Lecture on the benefits of humor https://www.harpercollins.com/authors/jamesmartin/

Managing stress through spirituality https://www.mayoclinic.org/healthy-lifestyle/stress-management/in-depth/stress-relief/art-20044464

A national strategy to prevent a clinician burnout pandemic https://www.nejm.org/doi/full/10.1056/NEJMp2011027

A selection of measurement and assessment tools to determine levels of stress and burnout https://www.proqol.org/

A summary of wicked problem characteristics and approaches to intervention https://hbr.org/2008/05/strategy-as-a-wicked-problem

This site offers general information on the concept of wicked problems including issues such as burnout http://tamingwickedproblems.com/

Zen philosophy and humor https://blog.sivanaspirit.com/sp-gn-importance-of-a-sense-of-humor-on-the-path/

Websites for the Classics

The following websites make available classical works in philosophy, psychology. and literature in their entirety. Useful examples are listed.

The Adventures of Huckleberry Finn by Mark Twain https://www.gutenberg.org/files/76/76-h/76-h.htm

The Courage Quotient https://www.optimize.me/philosophers-notes/the-courage-quotient-robert-biswas-diener/?mc_cid=7b80b616e2&mc_eid=%5BUNIQID%5D

The Enchiridion by Epictetus http://classics.mit.edu/Epictetus/epicench.html

About the Authors

For over 35 years, **Robert J. Wicks**, PsyD, has been called upon to speak calm into chaos by individuals and groups experiencing great stress, anxiety, and confusion. Dr. Wicks received his doctorate in psychology from Hahnemann Medical College and Hospital, is Professor Emeritus at Loyola University Maryland, and has taught in universities and professional schools of psychology, medicine, nursing, theology, education, business, and social work. In 2003, he was the Commencement Speaker for Wright State School of Medicine in Dayton, Ohio, and in 2005 he was both Visiting Scholar and the Commencement Speaker at Stritch School of Medicine in Chicago. He was also Commencement Speaker at and the recipient of honorary doctorates from Georgian Court, Caldwell, and Marywood universities.

Over the past several years he has spoken on his major areas of expertise—resilience, self-care, and the prevention of *secondary* stress (the pressures encountered in reaching out to others)—on Capitol Hill to members of Congress and their chiefs of staff and at Johns Hopkins School of Medicine, the U.S. Air Force Academy, the Mayo Clinic, the North American Aerospace Defense Command, and the Defense Intelligence Agency, as well as at Harvard's Children's Hospital and Harvard Divinity School, Yale School of Nursing, Princeton Theological Seminary and to members of the NATO Intelligence Fusion Center in England. He has also spoken at the Boston Public Library's commemoration of the Boston Marathon bombing; addressed 10,000 educators in the Air Canada Arena in Toronto; was the opening keynote speaker to 1,500 physicians for the American Medical Directors Association; spoken at the FBI and New York City Police Academies; led a course on resilience in Beirut for relief workers from Aleppo, Syria; and addressed care givers in China, Vietnam, India, Thailand, Haiti, Northern Ireland, Hungary, Guatemala, Malta, New Zealand, Australia, France, England, and South Africa.

In 1994, he was responsible for the psychological debriefing of nongovernmental organizations/relief workers evacuated from Rwanda during their genocide. In 1993, and again in 2001, he worked in Cambodia with professionals from the English-speaking community who were present to help the Khmer people rebuild their nation following years of terror and torture. In 2006, he also delivered presentations on self-care at the National Naval Medical Center in Bethesda Maryland and Walter Reed Army Hospital to those health care professionals responsible for Iraq and Afghan war veterans. More recently, he addressed U.S. Army health care professionals returning from Africa where they were assisting during the Ebola crisis.

Dr. Wicks has published over 50 books for both professionals and the general public including the bestselling *Riding the Dragon*. Among his latest books from Oxford University Press for the general public are *The Tao of Ordinariness*; *Night Call: Embracing Compassion and Hope in a Troubled World*; *Perspective: The Calm Within the Storm*; and *Bounce: Living the Resilient Life*. His books for professionals include *The Resilient Clinician* and *The Inner Life of the Counselor*. He is also Senior Co-Author of *A Primer on Posttraumatic Growth* and Co-Editor of *Clinician's Guide to Self-Renewal*. In 2006, Dr. Wicks received the first annual Alumni Award for Excellence in Professional Psychology from Widener University and is the recipient of the Humanitarian of the Year Award from the American Counseling Association's Division on Spirituality, Ethics and Religious Values in Counseling. In the military, he was an officer in the U.S. Marine Corps.

Gloria F. Donnelly, PhD, a national leader in nursing, is Dean Emerita, Professor Emerita, and founding Dean of the College of Nursing and Health Professions, Drexel University (1999–2016). Dr. Donnelly earned a BSN from Villanova University, an MSN from the University of Pennsylvania, and a PhD in Human Development from Bryn Mawr College. She is a fellow of the American Academy of Nursing and the

Philadelphia College of Physicians, the oldest medical society in the United States. Dr. Donnelly has served on many boards of directors, including Horizon House, Inc. a nonprofit serving the indigent experiencing mental disorders, of which she served as Chair of the Board. She currently serves on the board of Pennsylvania Health and Wellness, a health care insurance company and is a member of the national advisory board of the Nurses Service Organization, a professional liability company.

Early in her career Dr. Donnelly conducted assertiveness and stress management sessions for nurses and other health professionals throughout the United States as a member of a 3M-sponsored team committed to improving the lives and working conditions of surgical staff. This work led her to write a monthly series on assertiveness for *RN* magazine as well as a column through which she responded to nurses' work dilemmas. This work evolved into the publication of a book, *Coping With Stress: RNs' Survival Sourcebook*. Dr. Donnelly has held teaching positions at the University of Pennsylvania, School of Nursing; The College of New Jersey, formerly Trenton State; and Villanova University, College of Nursing. She led the development the School of Nursing at La Salle University and was the first dean of a newly configured School of Nursing at MCP Hahnemann University. She was Founding Dean of the College of Nursing and Health Professions, Drexel University, a result of the merger of MCP Hahnemann into Drexel in 2002. At Drexel, the college grew from 1,200 students in 2000 to nearly 5,000 in 2016 with 2,500 online students. Dr. Donnelly has been teaching online since 1999 in the Drexel University most recently in the Behavioral Health Counseling Program.

Dr. Donnelly is the author of five books and the winner of two *American Journal of Nursing* Book of the Year awards, the first for Sutterley and Donnelly, *Perspectives in Human Development*, and the second for Donnelly, Mengel, and Sutterley, *The Nursing System: Issues, Ethics and Politics*. With Doris Sutterley, she was a Founding Editor of *Holistic Nursing Practice*, a refereed, international journal originally published by Aspen, Inc. in 1979 under the title Topics in Clinical Nursing. Dr. Donnelly was appointed sole Editor in Chief of *Holistic Nursing Practice* now entering its 35th year of publication.

In addition to books, Dr. Donnelly has published more than 300 editorials and articles in leading nursing journals, including an invited career memoir in *Nursing Administration Quarterly* (Fall, 2017), which catalogues her own career transitions and cataclysms. She has also given hundreds of national and regional presentations on nursing leadership, problem-solving, transformation teaching, and the nuances of financial management of nursing programs for major nursing organizations such as the American Nurses Association, the American Association of Colleges of Nurses, and the National Student Nurses Association. For the past two years Dr. Donnelly has blogged for Drexel University Online and NursingCenter.com.

Dr. Donnelly has received numerous awards including the Alumni Achievement Medallion of Villanova University, College of Nursing; the March of Dimes, Lifetime Achievement Award; and the Pennsylvania Student Nurses Association Lifetime Achievement Award. Finally, Dr. Donnelly is also a stand-up comedian who has used her comedic talents for fundraising purposes and stress management for health care professionals.

Index

For the benefit of digital users, indexed terms that span two pages (e.g., 52–53) may, on occasion, appear on only one of those pages.

Tables and boxes are indicated by *t* and *b* following the page number